Luciana Gomes

Challenges for the integration of oral health actions

Luciana Gomes

Challenges for the integration of oral health actions

Between Primary and Secondary Care in Ilha do Governador, RJ

ScienciaScripts

Imprint
Any brand names and product names mentioned in this book are subject to trademark, brand or patent protection and are trademarks or registered trademarks of their respective holders. The use of brand names, product names, common names, trade names, product descriptions etc. even without a particular marking in this work is in no way to be construed to mean that such names may be regarded as unrestricted in respect of trademark and brand protection legislation and could thus be used by anyone.

Cover image: www.ingimage.com

This book is a translation from the original published under ISBN 978-613-9-62936-7.

Publisher:
Sciencia Scripts
is a trademark of
Dodo Books Indian Ocean Ltd. and OmniScriptum S.R.L publishing group

120 High Road, East Finchley, London, N2 9ED, United Kingdom
Str. Armeneasca 28/1, office 1, Chisinau MD-2012, Republic of Moldova, Europe
Printed at: see last page
ISBN: 978-620-7-75783-1

SUMMARY

I dedicate this achievement to God.

ACKNOWLEDGMENTS

First of all, to God, omnipotent, omnipresent and omniscient, who was with me at all times, enabling me and renewing my strength, in the most difficult moments, such as the many late nights I spent awake preparing this research.

To my family, especially my husband Thiago, whom I love and who supported and motivated me at all times, understanding my absences and having the understanding and patience to endure this battle; to my mother Lia, whose help and prayers were fundamental for me to achieve this victory; and to my father Ailton, who was also part of this achievement.

In an immeasurable way, to my dear advisor, Professor Dr. Carlos Serra, for his friendship, patience, dedication, wisdom and, above all, generosity in sharing all his knowledge on the subject and guiding me through this research.

To my dear Professor, Dr. Kâtia, who readily accepted to be part of my panel and was so generous in contributing her knowledge to the study, as well as always being so affectionate and supportive.

To Professor Dr. Marcos Senna, who also accepted to be part of my panel, giving up his private commitments, dedicating his time and knowledge in order to contribute to the elaboration of the research.

To all the teachers on the Master's Degree in Family Health who, in a particular way, helped build my knowledge, as well as generating admiration and love for the Family Health Strategy and Public Health, awakening in the students the desire to contribute, in some way, to the project of building the SUS, which is still in an evolutionary process.

I would like to thank the professionals from the units who took part in the research, including the coordinators of AP 3.1, for their patience, generosity and dedication during the interviews, as they were key players without whom there would have been no data to analyze. I would also like to thank the managers and directors of the health units who opened their doors with total dedication and promptness so that I could collect the data.

To my Master's degree friends, who helped me endure the hours of study without getting discouraged, always guaranteeing a "joke" in moments of great stress. In particular, I would like to thank three friends who have accompanied me most closely during this process: Friend Viviane, "Vivi", the "myth" of our class, our first teacher, who was always balanced, at the forefront of class decisions, and generous in sharing her knowledge with the rest of her classmates; my friend "Luisa Maria", whom I love for her energy and dedication in carrying out her tasks, no matter how great the challenges, and who was always my companion and "first-aider" to answer "all" my questions; and my friend Israel, whom I can't thank enough for everything he helped me with in this work; he really is a teacher par excellence, who will reach even greater heights.

To our dear course secretary, Ana Paula, who has carried out her work with such love and affection that it is reflected in a friendly relationship with all the students, who have in her a companion for all hours, helpful and dedicated to every request made and who gives everyone peace of mind even on the eve of the "epidemic" test.

To my boss, Marco Castanheira, my director, Jaqueline Urbani, and my head of human resources, Elizabeth, who were understanding and generous enough to release me from work to do this course, because without this possibility, this Master's degree, which has been my life project for years, would not have been possible.

To all of you, thank you very much.

So what should we say about these things? If God is for us, who will be against us? He who did not spare his own Son, but gave him up for us all, how will he not give us all things together with him, free of charge? Who will bring any accusation against God's chosen ones? It is God who justifies them. Who will condemn them? It is Christ Jesus who died; moreover, he is risen and is at the right hand of God, and he also intercedes for us. Who will separate us from the love of Christ? Will it be tribulation, or distress, or persecution, or famine, or nakedness, or peril, or sword? As it is written: "For your sake we face death every day; we are regarded as sheep destined for the slaughter". But in all these things we are more than conquerors through him who loved us.

(Romans 8:31-37).

SUMMARY

Introduction: The National Oral Health Policy - "Smiling Brazil" Program, considered a milestone in the history of public policies in Brazil, incorporating Oral Health Teams, expanding access and the implementation of Dental Specialty Centers (DSC), structuring elements of secondary care for the continuity of care initiated by primary care. In this context, effective referral and counter-referral systems are essential for integrating the care network and guaranteeing the comprehensive care provided for by the SUS and supported by the Federal Constitution as a right. **Objective: To** analyze how the articulation between primary and secondary care takes place and the perceptions and practices involved in this process, with regard to oral health actions in the district of Ilha do Governador, in the municipality of Rio de Janeiro. **Methodological design:** This is an exploratory, descriptive study with a qualitative approach, whose data collection instrument was a semi-structured interview script applied to the professionals involved in the RCR processes in oral health: dental surgeons from the basic units (seven interviewees), from the CEO (seven interviewees), professionals who operationalize SISREG (four interviewees) and the coordination of oral health in Program Area 3.1 (one interviewee). The data collected was processed using the Content Analysis technique. **Results:** The study revealed the existence of a formalized flow from Primary Care to the DSC, through the use of institutionalized clinical and referral protocols. However, there is a fragmentation of the oral health care line due to an insufficient supply of services and barriers to the integration of the network's points of care. These include deficiencies in the planning and organization of the supply of consultations in the medium-complexity area. In addition, there were weaknesses in counter-referrals, which were made using a paper guide, in communication between Primary Care and the Specialty Center, in technical support and in the continuing education actions carried out. There are also problems related to the lack of information systems, irregularities in the supply of inputs and maintenance of equipment. **Considerations:** Ilha do Governador's care network has promising prospects, given its project to expand primary care through the establishment of new units and the transformation of traditional primary care units into mixed units. In addition, the barriers described in this study can help the RJ Municipal Health System and the area's coordinators to make the necessary adjustments in order to guarantee users the right to continuity of care, operationalizing the integrality of care in their system.

Keywords: "Smiling Brazil". Comprehensiveness. Continuity of Care. Referral and Counter-referral.

1   Introduction

The proposal to reorganize the health system in Brazil was based on care networks that are categorized according to levels of complexity into primary (basic care); secondary (medium complexity or specialized care); and tertiary (hospital or high complexity).

In this model, primary care is responsible for resolving most of the problems related to community health, but when it is unable to resolve certain cases through its human and technological resources, they must be referred to other levels of complexity. In this way, in practice, there is a proposal for continuity of care, which begins at the first level of care.

At the beginning of the 21st century, public policies were characterized by the reaffirmation and expansion of the family-centered model. In 2000, Ministerial Order MS/GM No. 1444 was published, encouraging the incorporation of the Oral Health Team (ESB) into the Family Health Strategy (ESF). Also that year, the SB 2000 Project's oral health epidemiological survey was launched to assess the oral health conditions of the population, and was completed in 2003. The Descriptive Report of the SB Brasil Project revealed the precarious oral health conditions of Brazilians.

This survey led to the creation of the National Oral Health Policy - the "Smiling Brazil" Program, which is considered a milestone in the history of public oral health policies in Brazil, incorporating the ESB into primary care, thus contemplating the comprehensive care guideline of the Unified Health System (SUS). In this sense, the Program advocated expanding access to oral health at this level of care through the ESF and the Dental Specialty Centers (CEO), structuring elements of secondary care, to guarantee continuity of care, in addition to collective actions. In this approach, it is interesting to add the importance of a policy which, according to Cruz (2011, p. 181), has been interpreted as "social practices that express an intention to change an undesirable reality, which is done in action and which is embodied in the relationships between subjects".

Continuing the proposal to assess the oral health conditions of the Brazilian population that began in 2000, ten years on, the results of the National Oral Health Survey - SB Brasil Project 2010 - have provided one of the most complete diagnoses of the oral health of Brazilians to build a historical series, contributing to the evaluation and planning strategies of dental services. The International Dental Federation (IDF), with regard to oral health and diseases in the world, has shown that 90% of the world's population will have oral diseases throughout their lives (tooth decay, periodontal diseases, oral cancer and others); 60% of the world's population has access to oral care and 60% to 90% of school-age children have tooth decay and, as a result, toothache is the number one reason for school absenteeism in many countries (BRASIL, 2012a).

Although the burden of oral diseases has decreased in developed countries, periodontal complications have increased, especially in older people. Among the main risk factors are smoking, alcohol consumption and a diet rich in sugar, fat and salt, which contribute to various chronic diseases, including oral disease. According to the analysis of this research, prevention is fundamental and is done through proper brushing, the use of fluoride toothpaste and regular visits to the dentist and/or dental surgeon. Another point raised is that there are more than a million dental surgeons in the world using modern dental treatments with the aim of restoring oral function and aesthetics. Despite this, they are not equally distributed, leaving many regions unattended, especially the poorest and most deprived (MALTA *et al*, 2011).

According to the Ministry of Health, tooth decay continues to be the main oral health problem for Brazilians. The National Oral Health Survey, carried out in 2010 (SB Brasil 2010), presented the following data: at the age of 12, the rate of tooth decay was 56%; the average number of teeth affected by decay was 2.1, with variations by region; the need for dental prostheses in adolescents was 52%; and, among adults, there was a reversal of the trend: tooth extractions gave way to restorative treatments. In adults, the need for prostheses was reduced by 70% (BRASIL, 2012a).

Another important factor to consider is the fact that dentistry has undergone great technological and scientific development in recent years, but has not managed to effectively solve the oral health problems of the country's population. This justifies the high prevalence of diseases such as cavities and periodontal disease, which are still considered public health problems that need to be resolved (CARVALHO and SPYRIDES, 2013).

In this context, where the supply of services does not correspond to the real needs of the population, there are a series of difficulties related to repressed demand, waiting lines and guaranteed access to secondary or tertiary levels, since their needs are not fully met.

Despite the progress that has already been made, users are still faced with problems such as accessibility and the fragmentation of the services offered, which goes against the proposals for comprehensiveness laid down by the SUS and legally supported by the Federal Constitution, thus representing a citizen's right.

The principle of comprehensiveness, understood as continuity of care, is intrinsically linked to the articulation between primary and secondary care levels. For this reason, the motivation behind this research was to analyze the referral and counter-referral system (RCR), considered to be the main instrument created and used by the SUS to guarantee this principle in oral health, because when the integration of the levels of care of the health networks is not guaranteed by the effective functioning of the RCR, this system, which is one of the key elements in the reorganization of work practices, becomes a real critical node, causing damage to the integrality of care in general and, in particular, in oral health, compromising the consolidation of continuity of care in the SUS.

Thus, this study analyzed the flow of referrals and counter-referrals between primary and secondary care in the district of Ilha do Governador, in the municipality of Rio de Janeiro, a fundamental instrument for guaranteeing comprehensive oral health care.

In terms of the theoretical review, the work was organized into four parts. The first presents a brief account of the social and political construction of the SUS. The second addresses issues related to Primary Care (PC) and the configuration of care in Health Care Networks (HCN). The third part mentions oral health policies, with emphasis on the National Oral Health Policy (PNSB), implemented by the Smiling Brazil Program in 2004. The fourth part deals with issues related to the supply of oral health services and aspects of their regulation. The remaining items refer to the methodological procedures adopted in this research, the results and discussion and the final considerations, references, appendices and annexes.

2   Guiding Question

How does the link between primary care and the Dental Specialties Center work, and what are the perceptions and practices involved in this process, with regard to oral health actions in the neighborhood of Ilha do Governador, in the municipality of Rio de Janeiro?

3 Objectives

3.1 General objective

To analyze how the articulation between primary and secondary care takes place and the perceptions and practices involved in this process, with regard to oral health actions in the district of Ilha do Governador, in the municipality of Rio de Janeiro.

3.2 Specific objectives

- To describe the offer of oral health services in secondary care used by primary care units in the Zumbi and Bancàrios neighborhoods;

- To identify the criteria adopted by dental surgeons to refer users registered at the Zumbi and Bancàrios units to the secondary unit;

- Describe how scheduling for specialized oral health appointments works;

- Know the counter-referral flow from the Dental Specialty Center (CEO);

- Identify the strengths and weaknesses of access to dental specialties; and

- Survey the perception of the professionals involved about the process of consolidating integrality.

4 Theoretical Background

The items below have been developed in a simple and objective way, as it is not intended to theoretically exhaust the themes related to them. They are intrinsically linked to the object of this study, thus providing it with the necessary support for the development of this research.

It is worth emphasizing that the work is based on the constitutional principles of integrality, understood as continuity of care, and universality.

To this end, the theoretical review has been divided into four sections in order to contribute to a better understanding of the theoretical basis of the research proposal.

1ª Part: The Unified Health System (SUS): a political and social construction

According to Rodrigues (2014), the 1988 Federal Constitution (FC) enabled the political and social construction of the Unified Health System (SUS), albeit under the influence of particular and somewhat complicated historical circumstances for its implementation, as it was consolidated on the basis of a scenario of conjunctural changes, both national and global, from the late 1970s-1980s. In addition, the construction of this system was part of a broad process, in a social democratic model, of public policy changes between the state and society, making it possible to recognize health as a social right and a duty of the state.

The same author states that international circumstances were not favorable to the adoption of a comprehensive social rights policy, including health. In addition, from an economic point of view, the sharp rise in interest rates led to the so-called "debt crisis", which hit most Latin American countries and the former socialist bloc in Eastern Europe from the 1980s onwards, resulting in a large transfer of resources to creditor countries, especially the United States. As a result, in principle, there could not have been a more unfavorable international situation for the process of social justice contained in the 1988 constitutional text. However, even in the face of this adverse context, the approved constitutional text establishes the universal social rights of social assistance, education, health and welfare in Title VIII of the Social Order. It should be noted that internal changes accelerated the transition from the military regime to democracy and the implementation of social policies as a right of citizenship, despite the unfavorable international context.

On the other hand, this author points out that the development of the private health sector under public funding, in growing competition with the SUS, is an important factor and should be considered a challenge to its consolidation, in addition to the very weak base of support it has among labor unions, which are also attracted to private health, unlike what has happened in other public and universal health systems. In addition, decentralization to the municipalities would provide greater participation by society in health policies, with greater influence over public power, but it ended up making it difficult to organize the network of health services along regional lines for the exercise of citizenship in smaller municipalities, which are the majority in the country.

According to Fleury and Ouverney (2007), health policy should be treated as a social policy, i.e. one that focuses on individuals and the community. Like other social policies, health policy is subject to numerous determinants. It would be simpler, then, for every health policy to be aimed at improving the health conditions of the population, but there are other interests involved. They also state that, by considering health policy as social, one of the consequences is that health is assumed to be one of the rights inseparable from the condition of citizenship, but social policies are structured in different political and institutional directions that ensure access to a set of benefits for users of social protection systems. Furthermore, depending on the type of social protection adopted by a given country, access to healthcare can be a benefit, paid for in advance, a form of charity or even a right of citizenship, as in the case of Brazil.

In this way, this work will emphasize that the principles of universal access and comprehensive care, in the sense of continuity of care, are fundamental factors in solving health problems that cannot be solved by primary health care alone.

The right to public health is enshrined in the 1988 Federal Constitution, in Articles 6 and 196, as a social and fundamental right of the citizen and a duty of the state. Health, therefore, is inherent to being human, as is living a life with dignity. This condition is recorded in the Constitution in Article 1, Section III and reaffirmed in Article 196, Section II, which reads: "Health is the right of all and the duty of the State, guaranteed through social and economic policies aimed at reducing the risk of illness and other problems and universal and equal access to actions and services [...]" (BRASIL, 1988, p. 117).

With regard to the organization of the SUS, Article 198 states that "public health actions and services are part of a regionalized and hierarchical network", making up a single system, which is the SUS, organized according to certain guidelines, which are: "I. decentralization, with a single directorate in each sphere of government; II. comprehensive care, with priority given to preventive activities without prejudice to care services; III. decentralization, with a single directorate in each sphere of government; II. comprehensive care, with priority given to preventive activities, without prejudice to care services; III. community participation" (BRASIL, 1988, p. 117-18).

Law No. 8.080, of September 1990, the Organic Health Law (LOS), regulated the Federal Constitution of 1988 and laid down the conditions for the promotion, protection and recovery of health, as well as the organization and operation of the corresponding services. In Article 2 of this law, health is ratified as a fundamental right of the citizen, and it is up to the State to promote the conditions indispensable for its full exercise, while Article 3 of the LOS broadens the concept of health, pointing out its determining and conditioning factors, such as food, housing, basic sanitation, environment, work, leisure, among others, in addition to access to essential goods and services to prevent, promote and guarantee good health (BRASIL, 2011).

In its Article 7, the LOS also provides for the principles and guidelines of the SUS and adds that the public or private actions and services that make it up must be developed in accordance with the same actions provided for in Article 198 of the Constitution, following a list of principles. Among them are those directly related to the subject of this work, described below:

I - Universal access to all levels of care;

II - comprehensive care, understood as an articulated and continuous set of preventive and curative, individual and collective actions and services, at all levels of the system's complexity;

III - preservation of people's autonomy in defense of their physical and moral integrity;

[...]

VIII   - community participation;

IX   - political-administrative decentralization, with a single directorate in each sphere of government:

a) emphasis on the decentralization of services to municipalities; b) regionalization and hierarchization of the health services network; [...]

XII - the ability of services to resolve problems at all levels of assistance; and XIII - the organization of public services in such a way as to avoid duplication of means for identical ends (BRASIL, 2011, p. 115 - emphasis added).

In the legal sphere of health policy, the LOS and Law No. 8.142/90 regulate the right to health, pointing to the participation of society in the implementation of the SUS. Health policy must be recognized as a social right, given the programs that aim to ensure the health of the citizen and also the new models of care and techniques, based on parameters of access, reception, linkage and resolubility that prioritize preventive activities as opposed to the immediacy of the Brazilian health system, since health policy is based on a network of services, programs and projects aimed at providing good care for users (BRASIL, 2011).

However, the universal right to public health, despite being constitutionally guaranteed, has often been violated, especially with regard to comprehensive care, due to adverse contexts involving the Brazilian economic, political and social situation (BRASIL, 2011; SILVA, 2011). The current scenario in the city of Rio de Janeiro and the country in general is one of exclusionary public health rather than universal health, since the population that depends on the public health system is often faced with a lack of care. Thus, from a capitalist perspective, health will only be guaranteed to those who can "afford" it, which will probably increase the number of SUS users.

With regard to comprehensiveness, it can be said that this is certainly a permanent challenge facing SUS managers, as it is a question of guaranteeing continuity of care for users of this system. However, this principle will only be fully contemplated when all Brazilian citizens have access to basic health care and, according to their health needs, the guarantee of exams and consultations at the other levels of care that make up the network of hierarchical actions and services of the Brazilian health system in order to have their health problems resolved. Articulation between the levels of complexity of the network should be carried out through a referral and counter-referral system, an indispensable instrument for regulating the flow and counter-flow of SUS users.

According to Article 198 of the Constitution, the concept of comprehensiveness, with regard to healthcare, translates as "an articulated and continuous set of preventive and curative actions and services, both individual and collective, required for each case, at all levels of complexity of the system" (BRASIL, 1988, s/p). In addition, comprehensiveness demands that primary care has knowledge of the user's health needs, so that it can provide the necessary resources to meet them (STARFIELD, 2002).

According to Barbara Starfield (2002), comprehensive care ensures that services are tailored to health needs. When they are too limited, preventable diseases can occur or progress for longer, quality of life is at risk and people can die earlier. Thus, patients themselves recognize the importance of comprehensiveness and express dissatisfaction when it is not present. In addition, comprehensiveness is also assessed both by the availability of services that meet the common needs of the population, and by the appropriate use of these services to meet these needs.

The principle of comprehensiveness, according to Serra (2003), should be understood as guaranteeing the right of access to health actions and services at all levels of complexity and which is consolidated, in practice, in access to basic services and the construction of referral and counter-referral systems. Thus, the operational explicitness of this principle translates into a way of guaranteeing access and continuity of care.

According to Vilela (2010), accessibility to health services in Basic Health Units (UBS) is a very significant issue. With regard to comprehensive care, the author reports that "care bottlenecks" are considered difficulties and challenges; long waiting times; queues, including virtual queues; delays in test results, etc. In addition, the long waiting time for first access to the units is no longer the only problem, since other queues have been created as new demands have accumulated. The author also brings up the issue of computerized scheduling, which has generated "virtual queues".

According to Oliveira and Pereira (2013), comprehensiveness is one of the pillars of the SUS, enshrined in the Federal Constitution, and has four dimensions: the primacy of promotion and prevention actions; care at the three levels of complexity; articulation of actions and a comprehensive approach to individuals and families.

The first dimension goes against a health system that favors medicalization, presupposing a broader concept that does not restrict health to the absence of disease, but is capable of acting on its determinants, which are the social conditions in which people live and work. In this sense, intersectoral actions are strengthened since the health-disease process is the result of multiple aspects relating to all sectors of society. It is therefore up to the state to formulate social and economic policies that reduce social inequalities and improve living conditions for all citizens.

The second dimension takes integrality to guarantee access to different levels of care and therefore presupposes the existence of a network of services that must satisfy the individual through the integration of these actions. In the MS/SESUS/1990 document, the Ministry of Health (MS) describes integrality through a decentralized and hierarchical care model in which the integration of actions is guaranteed through RCR systems. Comprehensive care therefore depends on an articulated network at all levels of care, in a resolutive manner, with easy access.

The third dimension of comprehensiveness refers to the articulation of promotion, prevention and recovery actions, which have traditionally been developed separately. The last dimension concerns the integral approach to the individual and the family, relating to the creation of bonds, acceptance and autonomy.

2ⁿ Part: Primary Health Care, Health Care Networks and Access Regulation Systems

- Primary Health Care (PHC)

In this section, we will briefly and objectively discuss the importance of this level of care in the health system. In primary care, general practitioners work within the clinical limits of the specialties, trying to solve most of the health problems of the population under their responsibility. It is from this point that users are referred to the second and third levels of complexity in order to have their problems assessed or resolved. In this way, continuity of care, which is a constitutional right, can be achieved. However, in order to do so, we need to identify and overcome the numerous obstacles that still persist and prevent this principle from being contemplated.

According to Botazzo (1999), the UBS is the gateway to the SUS and should therefore absorb general demand, resolving approximately 80% of complications, as well as referring more complex cases to referral units or hospitalization. The UBS is also responsible for providing comprehensive care, enabling prevention and cure. However, in the reality of everyday life, people who need to access the system find multiple doors: some ajar, others closed and, for the most part, unequipped and disjointed.

According to Starfield (2002), primary care is considered to be an entry point for individual health care, as it promotes continuous patient responsibility and is a key component of a strategy to improve the effectiveness and equity of health services. However, this level of care is only one component of health care networks, albeit a fundamental one.

According to Giovanella and Mendonça (2008), the international historical context in the area of health, in 1978, led to the holding of the International Conference on Primary Care, in Alma-Ata, Republic of Kazakhstan (former Soviet Socialist Republic), which, in its final report, noted the responsibility of governments for the health of their peoples through sanitary and social measures, and reiterated health as a fundamental human right and one of the most important universal social goals, requiring action from other sectors, such as the social and economic, in addition to the health sector.

According to these authors, the costs of medical care, when using new technologies without adequately evaluating the benefits, gave rise to the term "appropriate technologies" because they are relevant to health needs, but with a high cost-benefit ratio. From this point of view, according to the Alma-Ata report, PHC should be based on appropriate methods and technologies that are scientifically proven and also socially acceptable, with access guaranteed to all, prioritizing community participation and the democratization of knowledge. However, it is not restricted to the first level of care, but is part of a permanent process which includes prevention, promotion, cure and rehabilitation.

Giovanella and Mendonça (2008) also report that, in Brazil, PHC entered the sectoral reform agenda in 1970, following the international movement, a period in which the economic crisis brought precarious health standards. Until then, health care had been spread by a pattern of consumption and high-tech services, controlled by the private sector and concentrated in metropolitan areas. Thus, the reorganization of basic services went hand in hand with the country's democratization process, which advocated the unification of the health system and the valorization of the first level of care.

In the 1980s, the selective approach was advocated for Latin America, through the use of a minimum basket of services, of low quality and restricted to the poor. In Brazil in the 1990s, primary care in the SUS sought a renewed conception, based on the concepts of universality, equity, comprehensiveness and the guidelines of decentralization and social participation. The term "primary care" was used, defining it as both individual and collective actions aimed at health promotion, disease prevention, treatment and rehabilitation at the first level. Thus, according to the aforementioned authors, first-level outpatient care, which becomes the user's first contact with the health system to solve most of the population's health problems, is considered a strategy for organizing the Brazilian health system.

The same authors report that in Brazil there was a movement to renew primary care, driven by international agencies (World Health Organization - WHO - and Pan American Health Organization - PAHO), which advocated broad and universal care in an integrated and horizontal approach, emphasizing prevention, promotion, intersectorality, participation of society and, finally, government accountability, reserving the following characteristics: first contact services; longitudinal responsibility; comprehensive care and coordination of actions. Based on this concept, services should be oriented towards the community, towards health needs focused on the family and with sufficient cultural competence to be able to communicate and also recognize the needs of the various population groups, emphasizing that there is a great diversity of care models that are the result of inter- and intra-regional disparities and also of the social inequalities that exist in this country, taking into account locoregional specificities.

In the 1980s, the Ministry of Health began experimenting with community health agents (CHAs), which, due to their success, led it to officially create the Community Health Agents Program (PACS) in 1991, with the aim of reducing maternal and child mortality in underprivileged regions of Brazil through professionals who lived in the community and were trained to advise families on health care (GRALHA & MORAIS, 2007).

As part of the proposal to strengthen PHC, the Family Health Program (PSF) was set up in 1994, with the family and community as its guiding principle. The PSF initially consisted of a basic health team made up of a doctor, nurse, community health agents and five nursing assistants (BRASIL, 2006a).

In 1996, the Ministry of Health issued the Basic Operational Standard (NOB 01/96) to define a new financing model for PHC. At that time, the Community Health Agents Program (Programa de Agentes Comunitârios de Saù) was merged with the Family Health Program (Programa Saù da Familia - PSF), in which community health agents contributed to carrying out the work of health surveillance and promotion due to their ease of communicating with people and their leadership. However, Ordinance No. 1886/97 approved Norms and Guidelines for the PACS and PSF, with the aim of creating incentives for both programs (GRALHA & MORAIS, 2007).

In 1998, the PSF came to be seen as a structuring strategy in the organization of the SUS in primary care and, in this sense, the transfer of the fund-to-fund financial incentives for the PSF and PACS began, i.e. from the National Health Fund to the Municipal Health Funds. In 1999, Ordinance No. 1,329 established the incentive bands for the PSF according to population coverage (BARBOSA, GALVÂO & MARTELLI, 2010).

Oral health was incorporated into the ESF in 2000, and the Ministry of Health also established a financial incentive for municipal reorganization of oral health care through Ordinance 1444/2000.

In this same ordinance, it was established that the area of operation of each PSF team should cover 6,900 inhabitants, and that only one Oral Health Team (ESB) could be implanted for every two family health teams (DIAS, 2006; NARVAI & FRAZÂO, 2008).

With regard to the broad and universal care in an integrated and horizontal approach, emphasizing prevention, promotion, intersectorality and the participation of society recommended for Primary Care, Giovanella and Mendonça (2008) state, specifically in relation to intersectorality, that this intersectoral action takes into account various aspects, such as biological, psychological and social problems considered collective, which are called determinants of health-disease processes. This is a condition for the realization of a comprehensive PHC, since health is inseparable from economic and social development, thus requiring coordination with other public policy sectors. The integration and coordination of care places PHC as a preferred gateway to guarantee access to the various levels of care, with mechanisms for reference and coordination of actions and guaranteeing continuous care, since integration, coordination and continuity are interrelated and interdependent processes.

In 2006, the Ministry of Health published the National Primary Health Care Policy (PNAB), which incorporated the attributes of primary health care, making it the preferred gateway to the SUS and a starting point for structuring the local health system. It is therefore understood, both individually and collectively, as a set of actions that promotes health, prevents illnesses, provides diagnosis, treatment, rehabilitation and health maintenance. In the form of teamwork, care is directed at populations in delimited territories, assuming health responsibility for them and considering the local dynamics of these populations, using high-complexity, low-density technology that seeks to solve the most frequent problems, in addition to being guided by principles such as universality, accessibility, coordination and continuity of care, establishment of a link, humanization, social participation, among others. Thus, the PNAB incorporated the principles and attributes of a comprehensive concept of PHC.

For Campos *et al* (2010), PHC should be one of the main gateways to the health system, which corroborates the analysis of other authors. However, much more is expected of it than just the function of guaranteeing access to the system, such as the ability to solve around 80% of problems while the remaining cases are referred.

The authors also report that PHC is usually less complex, with less sophisticated technologies and simplified technical qualifications. This tends to devalue the work and the professional. On the other hand, the organization of work in PHC is still confusing for the user and also for the system. Like the SUS in Brazil, the implementation of PHC is taking place in a very heterogeneous way and with unequal quality and capacity to resolve problems. We therefore propose an articulated network of services that expands the capacity to solve health problems, taking into account the following characteristics of PHC: 1) Accessibility[1] ; 2) Continuity or Longitudinality[2] ; 3) Comprehensiveness[3] ; and 4) Coordination[4] .

Ordinance No. 2.488 of 2011, issued by the Ministry of Health, approved the updating of the PNAB, bringing guidelines and norms for organizing primary care according to the Family Health Strategy (ESF) and the Community Health Agents Program (PACS). It also defines the organization of Health Care Networks (RAS) for comprehensive care geared to the population's health needs. One of the main strategies for integration was to set up computerized regulation centers to control flows and optimize resources, corroborating what is recommended by the Ordinance. However, its effectiveness is conditioned by supply, which, if insufficient, results in a waiting list, something considered to be the main problem for integration, contrary to what is recommended by the PNAB when it says that access to other levels of care should be under the right conditions, at the right time and with equity. Furthermore, the transfer of information is fundamental to the regulation and continuity of care, which is why electronic medical records are so important.

For Oliveira and Pereira (2013), PHC is recognized as a key component of health systems due to the evidence of its impact on the health of people in the countries that have adopted it, such as: greater efficiency in the flow of users of the system; more effectiveness in chronic treatments; better health indicators; greater efficiency of care; use of preventive practices and user satisfaction, in addition to reducing inequities in access to services and general health status.

The Family Health Strategy (ESF) was considered by the Ministry of Health to be a fundamental factor in the reorientation of primary care practices and the realization of the principles of the SUS at this level of care. Understanding its importance and operationality helps to reinforce the aim of this research, which is aimed at understanding and analyzing the continuity of care in the area chosen for this study.

Giovanella *et al* (2009) analyzed the implementation of the ESF as a tool for organizing the SUS, based on an analysis of the integration of Family Health (FHS) into the care network and

---

1Accessibility refers to the characteristics of the supply that enable people to access services, while access is the way people perceive accessibility. The concept of access brings the idea of non-restricted entry to health services and accessibility refers to the supply and production capacity of services and how to respond to the health needs of a given population (OLIVEIRA & PEREIRA, 2013).

2Longitudinality implies the existence of a regular source of long-term care, regardless of the presence or type of health problem. In international literature, the term "continuity of care" is used in a similar way to the word longitudinality, although these terms have conceptual specificities (OLIVEIRA & PEREIRA, 2013).

3Comprehensiveness is described in publications by the Ministry of Health as a principle contemplated through a model organized in a hierarchical and decentralized way, "with formal referral and counter-referral systems, whose guarantee of the integration of infrastructure resources is fundamental [...]" (OLIVEIRA & PEREIRA, 2013, p. 161).

4At the care level, coordination can mean "the articulation between the various health services and actions, synchronized and aimed at achieving a common goal regardless of where they are provided [...]" (OLIVEIRA & PEREIRA, 2013, p. 161).

intersectoral action, which are fundamental for comprehensive primary care. It should be remembered that, initially, the PSF, implemented in 1994, was aimed at covering areas of greater social risk. With the approval of the PNAB by Ordinance No. 2,488 on October 21, 2011, the scope of PHC was expanded and the ESF was reaffirmed as a strategy. Thus, from the perspective of being the gateway to a network of resolutive services for universal access, primary care should coordinate care and also implement comprehensiveness, the foundations and guidelines established by the PNAB.

Despite the great growth, according to Giovanella et al. the experiences reveal a great diversity of care models, a result of the inter- and intra-regional disparities and inequalities that exist in Brazilian society. Thus, the expansion of coverage has not always corresponded to the change in the care model advocated by the ESF. On the other hand, the professionals in the FH teams recognize primary care services as a preferential gateway, so that the population first seeks out the Primary Care Unit (UAB) when they need care.

According to Oliveira and Pereira (2013), the organization of primary health care services, through the ESF, prioritizes actions to promote, protect and recover comprehensive health, continuously contemplating practices and services that go beyond medical care and are based on the needs of the population, which are understood through the establishment of bonds between users and professionals. The ESF is centered on the family, perceived from its social and physical environment, as well as the living and health conditions of the population, allowing them a broader understanding of the health-disease process, with interventions that go beyond curative practices. In order to do this, professionals must have at their disposal a wide range of complex technological resources.

- Health Care Networks (RAS)

This section briefly presents aspects related to the reorganization of the health system into care networks and their intimate relationship with the subject of this work.

This model is characterized by health actions and services at different levels of complexity, but integrated, interdependent and without a relationship of subordination, since the difference between them is only in the use of technological resources. Another important aspect concerns the construction of RAS based on PHC, which is considered the gateway to the health system, responsible for solving most of its problems and, if this is impossible, ensuring access and continuity of care at other levels. This makes it essential to guarantee comprehensiveness for the HCN to be effective.

Mendes (2001) proposes a RAS in the form of integrated health systems, since fragmented systems are characterized by discontinuous care under the strong polarization between the hospital and the outpatient clinic, with hospital care being hegemonic. Integrated systems, on the other hand, are based on the continuous provision of services through various coordinated points of care and the integration of these points is achieved through powerful logistical processes.

For the author, the fragmentation of health systems is ineffective because they are essentially geared towards caring for sick people, since they do not emphasize promotion or prevention measures, nor do they take responsibility for the population. In this way, they are not focused on managing the risks to the population, they do not attend to people in their proper places and, as a result, they divide care and diseases into parts that do not communicate properly, causing the continuity of care to break down. In addition, these systems encourage the health care centers that have the greatest technological demand, which leads to the multiplication of technological resources. On the other hand, integrated systems are based on three basic pillars: evidence-based medicine, the economic evaluation of health services and the technological evaluation of these services. They are justified by demographic and epidemiological changes that point to a certain health situation.

Integrated health systems are defined as a reform of health systems through an integrated network of points of care that provides continuous and coordinated care to a given population at the right place and time, with the right cost and quality, as well as taking responsibility for the economic and health results related to this population, while the components of integrated systems are the management of the clinic, population risks and points of care (MENDES, 2007).

Mendes (2010) also addressed the crisis of health systems in terms of fragmentation and their focus mainly on acute conditions. The author reinforces the importance of the integrated systems that are the RAS, because they can "improve the quality of services, health outcomes and user satisfaction and reduce the costs of health care systems" (p. 2,297). According to this author, fragmented health care systems present isolated points of care that do not communicate, without guaranteeing continuity of care, considered to be a "health and economic disaster throughout the world" (p. 2.299), while the RAS, understood as polyarchic organizations, since they operate in a cooperative and interdependent manner, have a single objective, which is to provide comprehensive and continuous care, with quality and without hierarchy, since all levels have the same degree of importance, i.e. there is no relationship of subordination. This operationalization, however, requires a quality information system.

Network management is also discussed by Fleury and Ouverney (2007), who use the international theoretical discourse as a basis, as well as the regionalization strategy adopted by the SUS, to signal the emergence of a series of interdependent and multi-oriented networks. All these practices of administrative reform in health are not carried out randomly and must respond to an ethical foundation in the principles of universality, equity and comprehensiveness. As a result, one of the biggest challenges facing the SUS is that it is an unprecedented and open process, as well as reshaping the state machinery through new competencies and leadership. These authors also show how far Brazilian society has come in moving away from historical authoritarianism, in an attempt to turn towards a political management project that is more suited to the social, cultural and economic complexities imposed mainly by the country's own geographical characteristics.

According to Giovanella and Mendonça (2008), the first proposal for organizing health services was made in Britain in 1920, through the *Dawson Report,* which proposed a regionalized and hierarchical organization on three levels: primary, secondary and tertiary. In the 1970s, Canada, through a report by its Ministry of Health, showed the importance of disease prevention and health promotion, as well as government responsibility for organizing an adequate health system. This document was called the *Lalonde Report,* which established the relationship between health and living conditions, in particular environmental sanitation and nutrition, and criticized the biomedical model.

Corroborating the aforementioned authors, Rodrigues and Santos (2011) report that, at the beginning of the 20th century, the British doctor Bertrand Dawson proposed a classic concept of organizing health services, the so-called *Dawson Report*. It proposed the organization of preventive and curative health actions and services, integrated and based on community needs, with the primary level, with general practitioners and nurses, as the most important. In addition, actions and services must be accessible to the entire population, regardless of class, at all levels of complexity, integrated through patient referral. Thus, in Brazil, the organization of the system into health regions is represented by services and actions at different levels of complexity: primary, called basic care; secondary or specialized care; and tertiary, hospital or high complexity. It is worth emphasizing that the services at these different levels must work together continuously.

The aforementioned authors mention that a health services network involves many actors and elements, and is therefore highly complex. Its constituent elements are the points and the threads that connect them; the actions developed are the services made available and the policies directed at them, as well as human and technological resources and information, communication and logistics systems. The "points" are the units that carry out the health actions and services interconnected through the information, communication and logistics systems, considered the "wires". These information and communication systems are fundamental to guaranteeing user identification with the health card, as well as medical records, RCR systems, epidemiological information, authorization and invoicing of procedures, planning, controls and audits.

Thus, according to Rodrigues and Santos (2011), the information systems must be computerized and interconnected by the communication network through computers, telephones and other technological means, and the information must be available and always up-to-date. These communication systems must be agile, efficient, accessible to users, capable of establishing service priorities and controlled by management or regulatory centers. In addition, health service networks are only effective and efficient when they are guided by clear policies and defined health authorities, whose planning, control and evaluation bodies establish responsibilities and objectives for health services, based on epidemiological data from the region.

In this way, the resulting actions must be monitored and evaluated, with a view to intervening and making corrections if necessary. However, the SUS does not appear to be an effectively integrated system because, in a large part of the country, there are deficiencies in the information, communication and logistics systems, as well as in the planning and control bodies. This leads to difficulty in access for the population, queues, discomfort, anxiety and dissatisfaction on the part of the user, which goes against the rights of the citizen, who is the one who finances the service. Faced with this reality, it is of fundamental importance that problems relating to the health authorities or network management bodies are resolved in order for the system to function effectively.

According to Kuschnir and Chorny (2010), the organization of the integrated health system into care networks must guarantee continuity of care, as these systems are responsible for guaranteeing the right to health and regionalized networks as an instrument for expanding access and reducing inequalities. After all, this would provide health services for comprehensive care for the entire population of a region or territory, given that primary care would be the "gateway" to the system, with general practitioners, and would be linked to the secondary level with the offer of specialized services. Thus, cases that could not be solved at primary level would be referred to the other levels to which it would be linked.

The authors state that organization into networks would guarantee equitable access and comprehensive care for the entire population because the whole system should operate in a coordinated manner through referral mechanisms between the levels, supported by information and transport systems. In addition, they consider that the concept of hierarchization does not refer to a greater or lesser value between the levels, but rather to a complexity related to technological density and the importance of the first level should be emphasized with regard to resolubility based on the qualification of human resources, access to diagnostic and therapeutic means and links with the entire network.

Another consideration is the technical and political dimensions of national health systems that operate in networks, whose populations are defined geographically through regionalization. This is related to guaranteeing equal access to comprehensive care, as it involves power struggles and political decisions.

which are likely to hurt certain interests. For this reason, this model represents a major challenge, since the country has a peculiar combination of "triune federation with decentralization of health responsibility to the local level" (Kuschnir and Chorny, 2010, p. 2.315), which raises important questions about how to build regionalization, as well as the role and responsibility of each federated entity.

With regard to Oral Health, Mello *et al* (2014) evaluated the construction of the regionalized health network, focusing on Oral Health care, identifying difficulties and advances in its implementation, based on the network model suggested nationally by the policies that guide the SUS. In this context, it was found that the interaction of oral health care in the HCN in the regionalization process is sometimes disconnected from the set of relationships that make up the network, which is still being consolidated. On the other hand, the elements of the study indicate that the implementation of the regionalized care network is a condition for taking oral health care to a new level of care and assistance.

The aforementioned authors also state that in recent years, political and administrative measures, such as widening access to primary care, the inclusion of the ESB in the ESF, a focus on collective actions, the definition of lines of care and financial incentives, have strengthened oral health care as a public policy and promoted its expansion, qualification and visibility, constituting stimulating factors for the conception of the health network with oral components. Thus, with the implementation of the Dental Specialty Centers (DSC), the structuring of medium complexity dentistry provided more complex procedures and allowed continuity of care for users without interrupting the oral health care line. Thus, the structuring of a reference center was considered a milestone in the development of an oral health care network.

The aforementioned authors also point out that the effectiveness of the oral health network is influenced by the user's lack of knowledge of the system, especially with regard to the points of care, flows and limits of each level of care, leading to a negative evaluation. Thus, despite the efforts and progress made, there is a gap between what is laid down in the legislation and the reality experienced at the various levels, so that oral health care can be provided in a comprehensive manner. The work by Mello *et al* (2014) showed that the fractionated and autonomous action that prevailed until recently in the organization of oral health actions and services is not in line with the proposed RAS structure, which expects cooperative and integrated regional action.

As for strengthening primary care, it means more than expanding access; it means a strategy for organizing the system, reordering the resources that are made available to users. The ESB as a tool for reorienting oral health actions in primary care is fundamental to the network's composition.

From primary care, patients are referred to secondary and tertiary care, when necessary, in an integrated manner.

- Access Regulation Systems

In order to guarantee the integrality of the system organized through RAS, it should be noted that the effective functioning of the referral and counter-referral system (RCR) is of fundamental importance, as it must integrate the different points of care, guaranteeing continuity of care, which begins in primary care. The regulatory systems are responsible for guaranteeing access to tests, specialized consultations and hospitalizations at the most complex levels by referring patients. In Rio de Janeiro, this task falls to the Computerized Regulation System (SISREG), which is also responsible for oral health appointments and is therefore part of the subject of this research (BRASIL, 2006b).

The fully computerized SISREG was developed by the Ministry of Health during the period 19992002, representing the initial move towards the computerization of the so-called Regulatory Complexes. SISREG's objectives include:

- Equitable distribution of health resources to own and referred populations;

- Distributing available assistance resources in a regionalized and hierarchical manner;

[...]

- Allow referrals to all levels of care in the public and private provider networks;

- Identify areas of disproportion between supply and demand [...] (BRASIL, 2006b, p. 24).

According to Giovanella *et al* (2009), all managers are concerned with integrating the healthcare network. The strategy used to this end was the implementation of computerized regulation centers, with the aim of controlling user flows and optimizing resources. The implementation of SISREG has made it possible to immediately book specialized exams and consultations through a sufficient supply, the establishment of clinical priorities and the monitoring of waiting lists. The system makes it possible to monitor the user's journey, reducing the number of absentees, queues and waiting times, as well as making it possible to redistribute quotas between health centers, contract supply according to demand, analyze referrals and control agendas more impartially. It should be added that the effectiveness of integration is conditioned by supply, which is often not enough to meet the demand for specialized services, generating waiting lists.

Long waiting lists are seen as the main problem in integrating the network, according to both doctors and nurses in the FH teams. Managers, on the other hand, recognize computerized units and electronic medical records as a major challenge to integrating the network and guaranteeing access to specialized care, as well as the availability and transfer of information, as these are essential for regulation and continuity of care. When they are not present, the authors mention what they call the fragmentation of the system.

Another point raised by the authors concerns the purchase of specialized services from the private network so that they can make up for the shortcomings in the municipal supply. This, however, is not always a successful strategy in terms of the absence of some specialties as a result of the low remuneration in the SUS table. Another obstacle to be considered is the lack of policies from the Ministry of Health for medium complexity.

Gonçalves *et al* (2010) analyzed the evolution in the number of appointments and hospitalizations based on regulation. However, there is still a need for progress and consolidation of this process, which is considered to be a major challenge since it depends on the management capacity of each municipality to make the schedules of its services and professionals available. In fact, there has been progress in the care regulation system, but studies on this subject still need to be continued and deepened in order to take into account the particularities of access to health services in each region, in addition to measuring the impact and importance of a policy of logistical support for care networks.

According to Souza (2001 *apud* Gonçalves *et al*, 2010), the literature on the subject is still somewhat scarce, but it has been shown that many states have not fully taken on the role of regulating and coordinating the health system, as well as care and regional networks. To aggravate this situation, the reality of most of Brazil's small municipalities should be highlighted, because they have problems related to planning, regulation and the construction of care networks that are suitable for serving the population. As a result, from the point of view of quality, it cannot be possible - nor desirable - to guarantee the provision of medium and high complexity services in all municipalities.

3ª Part: Oral Health Policies in Brazil: a brief history

According to Ely *et al* (2009), public health policies in Brazil are related to economic policy and the historical moment. Following a chronological order, we present a narrative involving the main aspects of oral health policies in the country, relating them to the national situation.

In the 19th century, dentistry came to be considered a health profession in Brazil and, in the 20th century, from 1920 onwards, with the creation of the Retirement and Pension Funds (CAPs) for railway workers and then for seafarers, the first reports of a timid offer of oral health services in the CAPs appear.

In the 1930s, at the beginning of the Getúlio Vargas government, which lasted until 1945, the Retirement and Pension Institutes (IAPs) were created and oral health, offered to workers in various categories, was characterized by targeted curative practices, with priority given to pre-schoolers, schoolchildren and also pregnant women.

The 1950s and 1960s saw the creation of the Ministry of Health (1953) and the implementation of the Incremental School Care System[5] by the Special Public Health Service (SESP). The fluoridation of public water supplies began in Aimorés (MG) and Baixo Guandu (ES). In 1964, the III National Health Conference (CNS) was held, whose theme was the municipalization of health and was characterized by the advance of Dentistry in Collective Health, with the insertion of procedures for the prevention of dental caries through the use of fluoride in the National Public Health Plan.

In the 1970s, historical accounts record the population's discredit with public health (a crisis in the model) and, in the middle of that decade, during the military regime, the political opening intensified the movement for Health Reform and the Incremental System, which reached a national scale, providing dental care restricted to schoolchildren aged 7 to 14, through the SESP Foundation.

In the 1980s, the health reform movement grew stronger and popular movements intensified. Even though it wasn't approved, the PREVSAÙDE[6] , presented at the VII CNS, proposed that oral health should be one of the five main services offered by health units.

At the beginning of this decade, due to the expansion of dental care in the public sector, the Plan for the Reorientation of Dental Care (PRAOD) was created by the Consultative Council of the Social Security Health Administration (CONASP). During this period, several municipalities acquired dental equipment for primary schools and paid salaries to professionals through the Integrated Health Action Program (PAIS) at CONASP. In the public sector, oral health was marked by preventive actions, both individual and collective, using cariostats, sealants and fluoride to reduce the incidence of cavities.

In 1986, the 8th CNS was held, laying the foundations for restructuring the health system. In the same year, the First National Oral Health Conference (CNSB) was convened, bringing the conditions of dental care into debate and considering it an integral and inseparable part of the general health of the human being. During this period, the Ministry of Health created the Oral Health Technical Area and carried out the so-called *Brazil, Urban Zone,* the first epidemiological

---

5 From the 1950s and 1960s, and with the creation of the Ministry of Health in 1953, public oral health became institutionalized and was called "sanitary dentistry". This was the beginning of a system of care for schoolchildren in the public network, in a type of care called the Incremental System (MOYSÉS, 2013).

6 The National Program for Basic Health Services (PREVSAÙDE) was drawn up by an Interministerial Technical Group, with the aim of "restructuring and expanding health services, including sanitation and housing" (OLIVEIRA & TEIXEIRA, 1989 *apud* PUGIN & NASCIMENTO, 1996, p. 10). The program proposed "suspending new accreditation of private services and incorporating services provided by third parties into the network itself, subordinating other philanthropic or charitable institutions to strict state control" in order to extend basic health care to the entire population through "a single, hierarchical and regionalized network, under the control of the public network, seeking to reduce costs and rationalize care". PREVSAÙDE was not implemented due to pressure from the National Institute of Medical Assistance and Social Security (INAMPS) and other bodies (PUGIN & NASCIMENTO, 1996, p. 11).

survey of oral health in all Brazilian regions, the results of which revealed a worrying reality in relation to the oral health of the Brazilian population.

In 1988, the Federal Constitution was promulgated and the SUS was created. That year, in relation to oral health, we had, for the first time, a national program of a first specific policy for dentistry, which was the National Program for the Prevention of Dental Caries (PRECAD). In 1989, the production of fluoride toothpaste was regulated by the Ministry of Health.

The 1990s saw the regulation and national implementation of the SUS. In 1993, the II CNSB was held, with its final report proposing an effective inclusion in the SUS, guaranteeing access and equity of care in dental services. Following this, as already mentioned, in 1994 the PSF was created by the Ministry of Health based on the positive results of the PACS and in 1996, the SUS Basic Operational Standard (NOB SUS/96), aimed at strengthening the implementation of the PSF and PACS, instituted the payment of basic care on a population basis - the Basic Care Floor (PAB).

At the beginning of the 21st century, public policies were characterized by the reaffirmation and expansion of the family-centered model. Thus, on December 28, 2000, Ministerial Order MS/GM No. 1444 was published, creating the incentive for the official incorporation of the Oral Health team (ESB) into the ESF and regulating the ratio of one ESB to two FH teams. Also that year, the SB 2000 Project was launched in order to assess the oral health conditions of the population. For the ESBs, the incentives are differentiated into two modalities: Modality I, with a dental surgeon (CD) and a dental assistant (ACD); and Modality II, with a CD, an ACD and a dental hygiene technician (THD). In 2001, the actions of the ESB were regulated by Ordinance No. 267 of March 6. In 2003, the oral health epidemiological survey of the SB 2000 Project was completed and the SB Brazil Project Descriptive Report was published, revealing the oral health conditions of Brazilians. In addition, a new decree revoked the requirement to have one OHT for two FH teams.

According to the Portal da Saùde - SUS, dentistry was, for many years, on the margins of public health policies, and access to oral health was considered difficult and limited. There were few services offered by dentistry, so that the main treatment offered by the public network was tooth extraction. As a result, the view of dentistry was one of mutilation and of the CD professional as only a clinical practitioner (BRASIL, 2012b).

In 2003, in order to change this situation, the Ministry of Health launched the National Oral Health Policy (PNSB), implemented by the Smiling Brazil Program, consisting of various measures aimed at guaranteeing certain actions to promote, prevent and recover the oral health of the Brazilian population, as this is fundamental for the quality of life and general health of Brazilians. The main objective was to reorganize practice and qualify the actions and services offered by bringing together a series of oral health actions aimed at all citizens, extending free access to dental treatment by the SUS to the entire Brazilian population.

The program proposed the reorganization of primary oral health care, mainly through the ESB in the ESF; the expansion of access and the establishment of specialized care through the implementation of Specialized Dental Centers (CEO) and Regional Dental Prosthesis Laboratories (LRPD) and the addition of fluoride in public water treatment plants. Brasil Sorridente also articulates other intra- and inter-ministerial actions (BRASIL, 2012b).

In 2004, according to Ely *et al* (2009), the Ministry of Health's National Oral Health Coordination launched the guidelines for the PNSB, reinforcing the inclusion of the ESB in the PSF, the creation of CEOs and the organization of a national health surveillance system for fluoride content. With this, Oral Health was defined by the Ministry of Health as one of its priorities, especially after the launch of the Smiling Brazil Program as a government policy. That same year, the III CNSB (National Oral Health Conference) was held, focusing on access to and quality of oral health, in an attempt to overcome social exclusion.

According to Narvai (2006), the Final Report of the III CNSB/Brasilia, in 2004, reveals that oral health conditions are one of the most expressive signs of social exclusion and that tackling this problem requires much more than assistance measures carried out by trained professionals. What is needed are "intersectoral" policies that integrate preventive, curative and rehabilitative actions, focusing on health promotion and access for all citizens, as well as public responsibility on the part of the social segments and a governmental commitment involving the three spheres of the Brazilian state.

The document emphasized the importance of promoting equality in health care, reducing regional inequalities and expanding the supply of guaranteed health actions, as well as universal access for those most in need. In view of this, the same author says that it is hoped that the right to health in general, and oral health in particular, will become an integral part of citizens' lives and that access to all medium and highly complex dental services will be made possible.

According to Ely *et al* (2009), Ordinance MS/GM No. 648 was issued in 2006, regulating primary care and defining oral health actions at this level. The Health Pact was also launched, adopting two indicators for Oral Health: First Programmatic Consultation and Collective Procedures. The aim was to support action planning, as well as organizing access to services. In 2008, the professions of Oral Health Assistant (ASB) and Oral Health Technician (TSB) were regulated, changing, respectively, the previous names of ACD and THD.

- National Oral Health Policy (PNSB)

Narvai and Frazao (2008) analyzed the cruel face of health in Brazil, especially oral health, throughout its history in one of the chapters of their book called "Dental mutilation and perception of oral health". Through a historical retrospective of this problem, both in Brazil and in other countries, these authors reveal the main causes of this oral condition, while at the same time criticizing the professional practice of the DS and also the political, economic and cultural aspects of the Brazilian State, considering that in many regions and in several countries, the liberal orientation of the State provides a structure with a shortage of services, distributed unequally, in which professionals are trained to meet the needs of the consumer market rather than those of collective health.

It should be noted that the first oral health survey to include, in addition to all 27 state capitals, the inland municipalities of the five regions ("Projeto SB Brasil 2003") was carried out in 2003. The indicator used internationally for comparisons between countries is the DMFT (decayed, lost and filled - tooth unit) for the 12-year-old population. According to the classification adopted by the WHO, Brazil had a medium prevalence of tooth decay in 2003, with a DMFT of 2.78 (BRASIL, 2012a).

Based on the results of this epidemiological survey, which revealed the precarious condition of the Brazilian population's oral health, the National Oral Health Policy (PNSB) was established and implemented by the Smiling Brazil Program. This program understood this need, creating a strategy whose proposal is to set up a support network for OHT in primary care in order to provide continuity and resolvability to the problems encountered at this level. Thus, the DSCs are reference units for medium-complexity services, based on the guarantee of criteria identified for public access, based on an analysis of the risk and needs of the user and the implementation of the RCR. It can therefore be said that the rational use of levels of complexity makes the SUS productive and removes the obstacles that hinder the system. This guarantees comprehensive access for users and continuity of care (SILVA, 2009).

As for the Ministry of Health's Cadernos de Atença Bàsica, they arose from the need to organize health care in primary care, thus reorienting the care model in the SUS. It is known that, in order for the SUS to be effective, it is a *sine qua non* condition that primary care be strengthened, consolidating it as users' preferred contact with the health system. From this point on, access to other services must be guaranteed, which configures comprehensive care in accordance with the principles of the SUS.

In relation to Oral Health, Caderno 17 brings the PNSB guidelines, implemented by the Smiling Brazil Program, introducing a new model of Oral Health care, in an attempt to reverse a historical legacy, in which Dentistry walked away from other services, in order to integrate Oral Health actions with other health services (BRASIL, 2006a).

This booklet records the establishment of medium-complexity dentistry, based on the results of the 2003 Survey of the Oral Health Conditions of the Brazilian Population, which revealed the seriousness of the problems linked to the oral health of Brazilians and, in this sense, determined new actions to be carried out by the CEOs, created in all regions, in accordance with the respective municipal and regional health plans of each state.

In chapter 5 of this booklet, the recommendations for the RCRs are listed in order to organize the flows between primary and specialized care. According to these guidelines, DSCs should offer specialized oral health services with an emphasis on the diagnosis of oral cancer, specialized periodontics, minor oral surgery of soft and hard tissues, endodontics and care for people with special needs (BRASIL, 2004; BRASIL, 2006a).

The Smiling Brazil Program of 2003 was a milestone in the history of Brazilian public policies since the Brazilian Health Reform Movement, as it is based on the principles of the SUS. The program advocates the increase of oral health in primary care through the ESF, the implementation of CEOs (secondary care), as well as collective actions. The reorientation of the oral health care model, according to the PNSB, requires the use of epidemiology and information on the territory for planning, the use of health surveillance, with continuous evaluation of the damages, risks and determinants of the health-disease process.

In order to follow up and monitor the results achieved after the reorientation of oral health actions, based on the Smiling Brazil Program, a new epidemiological survey was carried out in 2010, the aim of which was to find out whether there had in fact been an improvement in the population's oral health conditions, and to reassess the actions and strategies. The results of the 2010 National Oral Health Survey, known as the SB Brasil 2010 Project, are also part of a historical process that has expanded and deepened since the SB Brasil 2003 Project, providing one of the most complete diagnoses of the oral health of the Brazilian population. The aim is to continue this process in order to build a historical series with the aim of contributing to service evaluation and planning strategies (BRASIL, 2012a).

The National Oral Health Survey 2010 (Projeto SB Brasil 2010), released on January 28, 2012 by the Ministry of Health, verified the situation of the Brazilian population in relation to dental caries, gum disease, the need for dental prostheses, occlusion conditions, fluorosis, dental trauma and the occurrence of toothache, among other aspects, in order to provide the Ministry of Health and SUS institutions with relevant information for planning prevention and treatment programs in the sector at national and municipal levels. The project is part of the Ministry of Health's health surveillance actions and is fundamental to the PNSB/Smiling Brazil Program, since its results will assess the impact of this program, identify problems and reorient prevention and care strategies, especially those related to the implementation of the ESF, aimed at primary care, and the CEOs, which are considered the structuring element of secondary oral health care (BRASIL, 2012a).

According to the WHO, Brazil went from having a medium prevalence of tooth decay in 2003 - DMFT 2.78 - to a low prevalence in 2010 - DMFT 2.1 - representing a reduction of 26.2% in seven years. Considering that the DMFT component refers specifically to untreated (decayed) teeth, the reduction was of the same magnitude, i.e. from 1.62 to 1.21 (BRASIL, 2012a).

It should be noted that the 2003 survey of the municipality of Rio de Janeiro showed that the DMFT of 1.4 at the age of 12 was better than the average for all regions of the country. This reflects consistent work to promote oral health, with emphasis on the Dentescola Health and Citizenship Program, as well as promotional actions in municipal health units. It also reflects the expansion of access and the qualification of the actions offered in primary care and medium complexity (BRASIL, 2012a).

According to the same source, there has been an improvement in oral health care in all Brazilian regions, except the North. Investment in the area rose from 56 million in 2003 to 600 million in 2010. There has also been a five-fold increase in the number of ESBs, so much so that 85% of municipalities have at least one team. As a result, the National Oral Health Policy (PNSB) has helped Brazil to join the group of countries with a low prevalence of cavities. To be in this group, the DMFT indicator must be between 1.2 and 2.6, according to the WHO.

The 2010 National Oral Health Survey analyzed the situation of Brazilian oral health and provided the SUS with relevant information for planning prevention and treatment actions at the national, state and municipal levels. Over the last few years, Brazil has learned to invest in reducing poverty and regional inequalities, and this is no different in the case of oral health, as shown by the significant 390% growth in ESBs, the creation of 865 CEOs; the qualification of 674 municipalities with laboratories for dental prostheses; the distribution of 72 million toothbrush and toothpaste kits; the expansion of access to treated and fluoridated water for around seven million Brazilians, culminating in a reduction in tooth extractions. This research report is the result of the work of SUS managers, researchers and workers to reorient the practices of professionals involved in oral health. Its results will contribute to equity in access to oral health, as well as representing an essential instrument for eradicating extreme poverty in the country, after all, expanding the RAS is fundamental for promoting citizenship (BRASIL, 2012a).

In Brazilian public services, oral health care, centered on curative/mutilative care, was modeled on the Incremental System imported from the USA (United States of America) by the SESP Foundation in the 1950s. In Brazil, priority was given to clinical care and the application of fluoride to students up to the age of 14, considered to be the most vulnerable and sensitive group to public health interventions, as well as being easy to approach due to their concentration in the school environment. In addition, emergency dental procedures were offered to adults and the elderly (AQUILANTE & ACIOLE, 2015).

According to the authors, with the emergence of the SUS, an attempt was made to break away from this "Sespian" model. However, only isolated experiments have succeeded in widening access, developing promotion and prevention actions and offering curative activities. In 2004, the PNSB - Smiling Brazil Program - was launched, proposing to reorient assistance by promoting health as the axis of care, universalizing access to services through the cross-cutting inclusion of oral health in the lines of care, as well as covering all levels of care (integrality) by setting up CEOs and LRPDs. In the public service, oral health care is no longer restricted to primary care for schoolchildren and pregnant women, as the PNSB expands access to services, mainly through the inclusion of the ESB in the ESF and also through the opening of the CEOs.

Almost a decade after the launch of the PNSB, the challenge still remains to make oral health care consistent with the principles of the SUS, and what has been observed in many municipalities is the continuation of a disease-centered model. However, the very positive gains, such as increased resolubility, comprehensiveness, interdisciplinarity, intersectorality, welcoming, bonding, accountability, humanization of care and working from the perspective of health surveillance, cannot be understated (AQUILANTE & ACIOLE, 2015).

Another factor to be considered, according to the same authors, is that the PNSB has made access to oral health care possible for many citizens, which has increased the demand for specialized treatment and, as a result, the DSCs are unable to absorb it satisfactorily. It's worth pointing out that a critical point to consider is the fact that consolidating the change will happen with a re-signification of the health work process and professional training.

4ª Part: Oral health in Brazil: services and access regulation

The oral health services offered in the public network start with primary care, which is responsible for health promotion, disease prevention and outpatient care. It should solve most of the problems, but when it exceeds its capacity to solve them, it has the responsibility of guaranteeing the user free access to the next level of care, which is carried out by the CEOs, reference units for medium-complexity actions in dentistry. Primary care is therefore responsible for guaranteeing continuity of care and coordinating health care actions.

- **Services offered in Primary Care in the Municipality of Rio de Janeiro**

The services offered for oral health in primary care, according to the Services Portfolio of the Municipal Health Department, are: a) Educational activities and group guidance; b) Oral hygiene instruction; c) Evidence and/or revelation of bacterial plaque; d) Supervised brushing; e) Typical application of fluoride; f) Clinical care outside the health unit; g) Home visits; h) Dentescola/PSE actions; i) Outpatient clinical care at the health unit; j) Tartarotomy or scraping of calculus; k) Restoration of anterior, posterior, deciduous and permanent teeth with amalgam, light-curing composite resin and glass ionomer cement; l) Periapical radiography; m) Clinical examination to identify lesions with suspected malignancy; n) Extraction of permanent and deciduous teeth; o) Referral to CEOs for medium-complexity procedures, such as: root canal treatment, severe periodontal treatment, periodontal surgery, complex extractions, panoramic X-rays, etc.p) Emergency care (RIO DE JANEIRO, 2011).

- **Dental Specialties Center (CEO)**

The Ministry of Health has created a strategy within the Smiling Brazil Program for restructuring dentistry based on regionalization, with the aim of improving access and also guaranteeing dental care in medium-complexity services, since there is a great deal of pent-up demand due to the greater coverage of primary care units. The treatment offered at the DSCs is a continuation of the care provided by the primary care network and, to this end, norms, requirements and criteria were established in order to set up and accredit these centers through Ordinance No. 1570/GM, on July 29, 2004 (BRASIL, 2004b).

The DSCs would be a medium-complexity reference for the networks of existing basic units and also for the ESBs incorporated into the PSF. Those that were accredited would receive funds from the Ministry of Health, according to Ordinance No. 599/GM, dated March 23, 2006, which defined norms, criteria and requirements for setting up and also accrediting the CEOs; Ordinance No. 600/GM, of the same date, and Ordinance No. 1572/GM of July 29, 2004 established the payment of dental prostheses in the LRPD. The implementation of the DSCs would work through a partnership between the municipalities, states and the federal government, with the Ministry of Health transferring part of the funds, while the municipalities and states would each contribute another part (SILVA, 2009).

According to this author, the CEOs are considered to be health establishments listed on the CNES and classified as Specialized Clinics or Specialty Outpatient Clinics. They are reference units for primary care and must offer services in accordance with the epidemiological reality of each region. They carry out clinical dental procedures that are complementary to those carried out in primary care and include oral diagnosis, especially the diagnosis and detection of oral cancer; specialized periodontics; minor oral surgery of soft and hard tissues; endodontics and care for people with special needs.

The transfers are made in accordance with Ordinances No. 599/GM and No. 600/GM, which establish the financing of the CEOs, according to each type: a) Type I, with three dental chairs, the amount of R$ 6.6 thousand is earmarked for monthly costs, in addition to R$ 40 thousand, in a single installment, referring to the costs of renovations, expansion of the physical space and acquisition of equipment; b) Type II, with four or more chairs, the monthly amounts of R$ 8.8 thousand and R$ 50 thousand are earmarked, respectively; and finally, c) Type III, with at least seven chairs, the costing resources are R$ 15.400.00 and up to R$ 80,000 (SILVA, 2009).

As for the implementation of LRPD, which are outsourced units accredited or owned by a municipality for the manufacture of total or partial removable prostheses, Ordinance No. 1572/GM establishes the payment of R$ 30.00 per production of each total prosthesis manufactured in these laboratories. As for removable partial prostheses, the amount paid is R$40.00/unit. The Ministry of Health transfers these funds directly to the municipalities or states that have accredited laboratories. Thus, in the author's opinion, there is no compromise of existing health resources, as they are considered "extra-ceiling" resources.

The shortage of specialized services raised the federal government's concern to encourage the creation of DSCs within the PNSB. Thus, there has been a growing advance in the implementation of these centers throughout the country, from 100 to 832 in the years 2004 to 2010, which represents an increase of 732%. Comprehensive oral health care requires valuing secondary care by strengthening and developing the RCR system. The difficulties in this regard are its obstacles, which need to be overcome or, at the very least, mitigated in order to guarantee that users' oral health needs are met (BORGHI *et al*, 2013).

However, according to the authors, in order to achieve the expected resolubility, secondary care must ensure that users have access to specialized consultations, procedures and exams. However, these services are just one of the aspects of the current PNSB and these centers are one of the fronts of the Smiling Brazil Program, and the flow of care consists of primary care professionals being responsible for the first care of the patient and also for referring more complex cases to the DSCs.

- **Regulating Access to Services**

The consolidation of the principles of universal access and comprehensive care of the SUS, in the sense of continuity of care, which underpin this research, necessarily involves the linking of the Basic Health Units with the other levels of complexity through a well-structured RCR system. In this case, primary care guarantees access to the next higher level of care when it is unable to solve the user's health problems. The RCR system will act as a link between the user and the other levels of care, allowing them to traverse the entire health system, at all levels, according to their needs, and always return to the point of origin, which is primary care.

Serra (2003), quoting Giovanella *et al* (2002), shows that comprehensiveness encompasses five dimensions: the human being and not the disease as the center of care; a view of the human being or group as a whole; assistance offered at the various levels of care; differentiated treatment for those in unequal situations; and interference in the general living conditions of the population. In this way, it can be inferred that integrality is related to the instruments of reference and counter-reference (RCR) and is articulated in a hierarchical and regionalized system, with continuity of care as its guiding principle, which guarantees universal and equal access for users to primary care and other levels, according to the needs of each individual.

Thus, in order to guarantee the integrality of the system organized through HCN, the effective functioning of the RCR system is of fundamental importance, as it is the system that guarantees integration between the different points of care and continuity of care, which begins in primary care. The regulatory systems are responsible for guaranteeing access to tests, specialized consultations and hospitalizations at the most complex levels by referring patients. In Rio de Janeiro, this task falls to the Computerized Regulation System (SISREG), which is also responsible for oral health appointments and is therefore part of the subject of this research (BRASIL, 2006b).

The fully computerized SISREG was developed by the Ministry of Health during the period 19992002 to computerize the central regulation system, representing the initial move towards the computerization of the so-called Regulatory Complexes. SISREG's objectives include:

- Equitable distribution of health resources to own and referred populations;

- Distributing available assistance resources in a regionalized and hierarchical manner;

[...]

- Allow referrals to all levels of care in the public and private provider networks;

- Identify areas of disproportion between supply and demand [...] (BRASIL, 2006b, p. 24).

According to Giovanella *et al* (2009), it is the concern of all managers to integrate the care network and, specifically, primary care with medium-complexity care, with the aim of clarifying the diagnosis quickly so that the user's health conditions can be resolved and monitored. To this end, the strategy used was to set up computerized regulation centers in order to control flows and optimize resources. The implementation of SISREG has made it possible to immediately book specialized exams and consultations by providing a sufficient supply, establishing clinical priorities and monitoring waiting lists. The system makes it possible to monitor the user's journey, reducing the number of absentees, queues and waiting times, as well as making it possible to redistribute quotas between health centers, contract supply according to demand, analyze referrals and control agendas more impartially. It should be added that the effectiveness of integration is conditioned by supply, which is often not enough to meet the demand for specialized services, generating waiting lists.

According to the authors, long waiting lists are the main problem in integrating the network, as assessed by both doctors and nurses in the FH teams. Managers recognize computerized units and electronic medical records as a major challenge to integrating the network and guaranteeing access to specialized care, as well as the availability and transfer of information, as these are essential for regulation and continuity of care.

However, when these conditions are not present, the so-called fragmentation of the system inevitably occurs. Another point raised by the authors concerns the purchase of specialized services from the private network so that they can make up for the shortcomings in the municipal supply. This, however, is not always a successful strategy when it comes to the absence of some specialties, due to the low remuneration of the SUS table. Another obstacle to be considered is the lack of policies from the Ministry of Health for medium complexity.

As a strategy adopted by the Ministry of Health (MS), the Family Health Program (PSF) is capable of reviving the principles of the SUS, as well as reordering and restructuring the system's gateway to a greater degree of organization and resolution at the various levels of care. However, in order to achieve full universality, the Family Health Units (USF) must be articulated with the other levels of complexity, which can only be achieved through a well-structured RCR system that can guarantee continuity of care in order to solve the user's health needs. The RCR system should be the link between the user and the other levels of care, allowing them to go through the whole system according to their needs and always return to the point of origin, which is primary care (SILVA, 2009).

Gonçalves *et al* (2010) analyzed the evolution in the number of appointments and hospitalizations based on regulation. However, there is still a need to advance and consolidate this process, which is considered to be a major challenge since it depends on the management capacity of each municipality to make the schedules of its services and professionals available. In fact, there has been progress in the care regulation system, but studies on this subject still need to be continued and deepened in order to take into account the particularities of access to health services in each region, in addition to measuring the impact and importance of a policy of logistical support for care networks.

According to Souza (2001 *apud* Gonçalves *et al*, 2010), the literature on the subject is still somewhat scarce, but it can be seen that many states have not fully taken on the role of regulating or coordinating the health system and the care and regional networks. To make matters worse, the reality of most of Brazil's small municipalities must be highlighted. They have problems related to planning, regulation and the construction of care networks that are suitable for serving the population. As a result, from the point of view of quality, it cannot be possible - nor desirable - to guarantee the provision of medium and high complexity services in all municipalities.

Serra and Rodrigues (2010) consider that the concept of comprehensive health care, the first established in the 1988 Federal Constitution as the second guideline of the SUS, and comprehensive care as one of its principles by the LOS, refer to the right of users to access the actions of the different levels of complexity, with defined and spatially organized flows in order to ensure continuity of care in units located close to the citizens. The integration of health networks is guaranteed by the effective RCR system, which establishes the mutual referral of patients between the different levels of complexity, since the Ministry of Health itself defines this system as one of the key elements in the reorganization of work practices.

Thus, integration involves various interrelated aspects, such as: "service regulation; conditions of access to services; clinical management processes; human resources; information and communication systems and logistical support". All of these aspects are considered critical to guaranteeing the proper functioning of the RCR, and its inadequate functioning causes damage to the integrality and continuity of care, which are fundamental to the consolidation of the SUS (SERRA E RODRIGUES, 2010, p. 3.580).

In a study carried out by the same authors, among the results obtained that hinder patient access and the proper functioning of RCR systems in the areas surveyed are:

(1) limited supply of consultations and exams; (2) non-existent or precarious counter-referrals; (3) poorly organized regulation activities; (4) low use of clinical protocols for referrals; (5) precarious information and communication systems; (6) significant political influence on the management of the units; (7) great diversity in the names of the health units and multiplicity of the range of services on offer (SERRA & RODRIGUES, 2010, p. 3.577). 3.579).

The authors consider that one of the main critical points of the system is the RCR, but at the same time it is one of the most important parts for the viability and maintenance of the SUS. This system operates by referring users to different levels of complexity, and it is only by guaranteeing access to exams, specialized consultations and hospitalizations that comprehensive care becomes possible. For this reason, a maximum degree of resolubility must be achieved at each level of the system, since referring patients without exhausting all the technical possibilities and resources available strangles the more complex levels and makes the system inefficient.

According to Silva (2009), RCR should be understood as part of a "puzzle", which leads us to say that the rational use of levels of complexity makes the SUS productive and undoes the knots that hinder the system, as it "fits the pieces together", facilitating comprehensiveness in terms of user access and continuity of care.

Serra and Rodrigues (2010) evaluated the RCR system in USFs in the municipalities of Duque de Caxias (Metropolitan Region/RJ) and Rio de Janeiro, analyzing the resolubility of the PSF, under the support of the secondary level to carry out specialized consultations and exams, which depends on the proper functioning of the system. It is known that the PSF is a strategy for reorganizing the SUS and reorienting PHC, reviving fundamental principles and guidelines. The concept of comprehensiveness, provided for in the 1988 Constitution as a guideline and as a principle in the LOS, as in both, refers to the right of users to access the actions of the different levels of complexity, with spatially defined and organized flows to ensure continuity of care in units located as close to the citizens as possible. Thus, the units at each level of care must be sized in such a way as to guarantee the provision of services of sufficient quantity and quality.

The integration of health networks is guaranteed by the effective system of RCR, which establishes the mutual referral of patients between the different levels of complexity of the services. The Ministry of Health itself defines this system as one of the main elements in the reorganization of working practices, since integration involves several interrelated aspects, such as regulating services; clinical management processes; conditions of access to services; human resources; information systems, communication and logistical support. All of these are considered critical elements in ensuring a well-functioning RCR system.

The authors report that, since the 20th century, there has been an increase in health costs and the main contributing factors have been diagnostic and therapeutic procedures, associated with new specialties; the intense technological incorporation of equipment and drugs; the increase in population longevity and the growth of chronic conditions. As a result, access to all levels of the system has become a problem, since there has been no planning of the supply of specialized consultations and exams based on the health needs of the population. In addition, there was little control by managers over the provision of services by secondary units whose heads are politically appointed.

The main problems with referrals, according to the same authors, are the lack or precariousness of counter-referrals, the limited supply of consultations and exams and the poor organization of regulation, as well as the difficulty of access due to financial problems, such as the cost of tickets. Another important finding for the authors was the variation in nomenclatures, which can make it difficult for users to be identified and referred. With regard to information systems, neither of the two areas studied had implemented the SUS Card or had electronic medical records and systems for scheduling appointments and specialized exams, and this hampers the effective functioning of the RCR.

With regard to logistical support for the USFs, there was a frequent shortage of medicines, which compromises the control of chronic diseases, as it results in complications and increased costs. The authors also found poor maintenance and calibration of biomedical equipment, leading to errors in diagnosis and improper prescriptions, with serious consequences for patients.

The study exposed some of the operational deficiencies necessary for the proper functioning of the RCR between PHC and the other levels of complexity, in all the aspects considered. The management bodies do not have effective control over the secondary units due to a lack of planning, regulation and political appointment of the heads of these units. The supply of services continues to be geared towards meeting spontaneous demand rather than the real needs of the population, based on epidemiological criteria. In addition, the random spatial distribution of the units and their inadequate sizing in relation to demand were also evidence of this lack of planning (SERRA & RODRIGUES, 2010).

With regard to clinical management, the authors found a lack or deficiency of clinical protocols and referrals that were poorly supported by clinical protocols and guidelines. This reveals the need for continuing education programs as well as adaptation to the local reality. There was also a lack of technical support for the teams, which makes it difficult for professionals to make decisions and increases the number of referrals. Counter-referrals were almost non-existent.

With regard to human resources, it was observed that there are professionals without appropriate training; lack of training for the job; precarious permanent education; irregular employment contracts; isolation of professionals working in small units and without technical support. In addition, the information and communication systems are precarious, as there is a lack of networked telephones and computers, electronic medical records and systems for scheduling appointments and exams. For this reason, the most commonly used means of RCR is through paper forms.

Thus, the study by the aforementioned authors provides relevant information for this research and, through it, we can understand the reduced resolubility of the Program, which has implications for the health of the population. In addition, the inadequate functioning of the RCR, observed in the study, causes damage to the integrality and continuity of care, which are fundamental for the consolidation of the SUS.

Pimentel *et al* (2010) observed, in a study on the referral of patients to medium and high complexity services, some difficulties both in the lack of agreements for certain municipal services and in the evident accumulated demand, especially for the specialty of endodontics. These authors reinforce these findings when they state that if the needs of the local service are not resolved, there is no RCR scheme and the problems remain unsolved, as users cannot afford treatment in the private network. In this way, dentistry is unable to solve the oral problems of its population because of the huge demand that has built up.

The authors also report that the faster and more reliable the referral, the greater the chances of the patient following the correct referral flow. According to the Caderno da Atença Bàsica - Saùde Bucal, referrals should be made using RCR forms, accompanied or not by complementary exams and X-rays.

Another important point is the follow-up of the referred patient, who often does not return to the unit of origin for follow-up and/or completion of treatment. Ideally, once the treatment is finished, the patient should be sent back to the health unit of origin to complete the treatment and maintenance, with the counter-referral form duly filled in, which should include the identification of the professional, the diagnosis and the treatment carried out (PIMENTEL *et al,* 2010).

Vilarinho, Mendes and Prado Jùnior (2007) reported in studies carried out in Teresina (PI) that the DCs did not have a detailed knowledge of how to solve the problems referred to the referral services, and also that the only CEO in the municipality at the time was unable to fully meet the demand, thus leading to a discontinuity of dental care at the secondary and tertiary levels.

In addition to the high demand, the authors report that the low supply capacity of secondary and tertiary care services compromises the proper establishment of oral health RCR systems. In the dental sector, the expansion of the secondary and tertiary care network has not kept pace with the growth in the supply of primary care services.

According to Borghi *et al* (2013), in order to achieve comprehensive oral health care, it is necessary to organize the "gateway" to this system, i.e. primary care and, above all, its interconnection with secondary care. It was observed that there was a flow of care from primary care to secondary care in oral health, and they were satisfied with the service. However, counter-referral was significantly deficient, considering that the majority of patients did not return to primary care. Considering the principle of comprehensiveness and the construction of care networks in the SUS, secondary care can reflect the resolubility of primary care by supporting the organization of oral health actions and services in the context of medium complexity. Comprehensiveness in oral health, as well as being a principle of the SUS, is a constitutional right guaranteed to every citizen and, in order to achieve it, the system must function correctly.

In recent decades, there has been an emphasis on health promotion and the strengthening of primary oral health care through actions carried out in the USF and UBS. Thus, four important characteristics were defined for the interconnection between primary and secondary dental care: 1) Indiscriminate and unhindered access to specialized care after referral; 2) A referral system in which all services unavailable in primary care are offered in specialized care; 3) Efficient and appropriate referral with counter-referral to primary care at the end of specialized treatment; and 4) Easy return to secondary care whenever necessary (BORGHI *et al*, 2013).

For the authors, most dental care in the SUS has been restricted almost solely to primary care and with a large pent-up demand, reflecting the country's social inequalities in the use of dental services. In 2000, according to the Ministry of Health, secondary care had low percentages, only 3.3% within the scope of dental procedures. The lack of specialized services compromises the efficiency of the RCR in Oral Health. These facts culminated in the federal government's concern to encourage the creation of CEOs within the PNSB.

The concept of service provision, implicit in the definition of coverage, means that these services are accessible to the community and meet their health needs. However, the mere existence or availability of a service does not guarantee accessibility. For this reason, according to the authors, it is necessary to subdivide this concept into geographic accessibility - distance, travel time and means of transportation; financial accessibility - payments or contributions for the use of services should not represent obstacles; cultural accessibility - there should be no conflict between the technical and administrative standards of the services and the habits, cultural patterns and customs of the communities; and functional accessibility - services should be provided in a timely and continuous manner, available at all times in order to meet real demand under a referral system that ensures easy access.

According to the same authors, the non-return of patients from the DSC is an obstacle to comprehensiveness, as there is no continuity of care. The specialist professional must make an effort to provide counter-referrals and, above all, to inform patients of the importance of returning to conclude the case. For example, the main causes of treatment abandonment were the inability to take time off work, the length of treatment and causes external to the service, such as illness, pregnancy and moving house. It should be noted that the impact of oral health actions in primary care has made clear progress in terms of universality, equity and comprehensiveness. This analysis contributes to the evaluation of the organization of primary care, considering that comprehensive care is achieved through the coordination of care by PHC integrated into the network at the other levels of care, from access to the resolution of existing health needs.

However, it is clear that efforts need to be made to organize the demand for primary care in order to guarantee access for these patients returning from secondary care, helping to monitor the health care of users who pass through the municipality's oral health care network. Thus, adjustments need to be made, especially from the point of view of the management of the units and their communication with patients. It is essential to reflect on the organization of the counter-referral of patients to primary care in order to guarantee the integrality of oral health care, a key factor in ensuring the longitudinality of care and the quality of care (BORGHI *et al*, 2013).

The authors also report that regionalization proposes comprehensive access, the reduction of inequalities and decentralized management. In order for it to be implemented, municipal health systems had to be organized in such a way as to provide comprehensive health care, in accordance with the definition of comprehensive care contained in the 1988 Constitution, in its Article 7, Item II, which is comprehensive care understood as an articulated and continuous set of actions and services that are preventive and curative, both individual and collective, and obeying the needs of each case at all levels of the system's complexity.

Thus, for the authors, one of the major critical points of the system is the RCR, while at the same time it is one of the points of fundamental importance for the viability and maintenance of the SUS, since it is from its structuring that the referral of patients between levels of care becomes possible. Structuring the responsibilities and attributions of each sphere of competence is necessary since referring clients to other levels of complexity without exhausting diagnostic possibilities is a mistake in health care.

Therefore, there should be a maximum degree of resolvability at each level of the system, where dealing with the client without exhausting the technical possibilities and resources available makes the system inefficient and bottlenecks the more complex levels. ABS is the level at which the degree of problem resolution should be approximately 80%; therefore, efforts should be focused on improving the quality of the teams working at this level. The opposite means overloading the levels of the system and creating unnecessary knots in the care network (BORGHI *et al*, 2013).

However, in order to achieve such resolubility, the same authors report that the secondary level of care must ensure that users have access to specialized consultations and exams. This perspective of an integrated health system is represented by a network of care with multiple dimensions of integration between the different subsystems in which the determination of levels of complexity for the adequacy and expansion of the primary network should be based on the degree of differentiation of the activities carried out at each of the levels established, which are: primary, secondary and tertiary.

However, the Brazilian health system, which has emphasized the principles of regionalization since the 1980s, is still in a precarious state of organization, unable to guarantee continuity of care, thus generating duplication of work and costs, as well as a lot of inconvenience for users. The Smiling Brazil Program understood this need and created a strategy that aims to create a support network for OHT in primary care, in order to provide continuity and resolvability to the problems encountered at this level and, in this way, the DSCs become reference units with medium complexity services. It is based on the guarantee of publicly identified access criteria, included in the care network, based on risk analysis and user needs, with the implementation of RCR protocols (BORGHI *et al*, 2013).

- Oral Health Care Network: Challenges for Integration

Santos and Assis (2006) analyzed oral health practice in the PSF in Alagoinhas/BA (2001-2004), looking at the devices that guide comprehensive oral health care: linkage, reception, autonomy, accountability and resolubility. The results show that practice is organized through individual and collective actions, built on a repressed demand; care is fragmented, with excessive emphasis on technique and specialty, whose axis is ordered by the medical-centered model, with limited resolubility; welcoming is manifested through a tense and conflicting relationship, but with the potential to build alternatives for change; the bond and autonomy intersect in the rescue of the worker-user relationship and in the meeting of their potential, making it possible to horizontalize knowledge, strengthen ties and consolidate affections.

In short, oral health practice is full of conflicts and contradictions and is a potential tool for changing work processes, coexisting with the old (fragmentation) and the new (integrality) in an unfinished process, still under construction, according to the authors cited. Comprehensive care, defined as the articulation of health promotion, prevention and treatment actions in the individual and collective spheres, implies a paradigm shift in professional oral health practices, which have historically been based on individual clinical care. The continued centralization of clinical practices is justified by the repressed demand in the area of oral health.

According to Narvai and Frazao (2008), dental care in Brazil, despite all the advances, is characterized by being predominantly liberal, through direct disbursement or through health plans. Oral health, treated as a commodity, not only alienates the DS, but also empties the meaning of the practice itself, leading to restricted access and fragmented actions.

For these authors, overcoming the "procedure-centered" model, valuing therapeutic diversity, including the user in the care process and integrating promotion, prevention, cure and rehabilitation requires changes in the educational project. The authors talk about the paradigmatic nature of the implementation of the SUS and the subsequent prioritization of primary health care as the service of first contact through the ESF. The achievements of the Health and Oral Health Conferences in the Collective Oral Health Movement should also be highlighted, marking a break with the liberal, corporatist and exclusionary nature of dentistry.

Chaves *et al* (2010) carried out a study with the aim of analyzing factors related to comprehensive oral health care in DSCs according to the guiding principles of the PNSB. The author concluded that younger users, with easier geographical access and a need for endodontic services, were more likely to receive comprehensive care. The implementation of DSCs in municipalities where primary health care is not adequately structured is not recommended, since secondary care would be meeting free demand and performing basic procedures, thus not fulfilling the principle of comprehensiveness.

Bulgarelli *et al* (2013) carried out a study to evaluate the models of primary oral health care in the municipality of Marilia/SP using information on secondary dental care, according to the Principle of Comprehensiveness. It was concluded that, regardless of the organizational model of the local primary care services - traditional or ESF - the results regarding secondary dental care are similar in terms of access, absences, abandonment and resolubility. It is important to evaluate oral health care models in order to guide the planning and execution of actions at municipal level, which is essential for building a more resolute public dentistry, with greater efficiency and quality, making the principles of the SUS a reality, especially in relation to integrality in health care networks.

Aquilante and Aciole (2015) show that some studies have identified DCs restricted to basic outpatient clinical care, such as exodontia, plaque detection, dietary guidance, typical fluoride application, restorations, oral hygiene guidance and basic periodontal procedures, while Oral Health Assistants are focused on activities considered conventional, such as CD instrumentation, disinfection and sterilization of materials and instruments, without prioritizing collective actions such as home visits, meetings with the community and health prevention and promotion actions.

Given this reality, the need for professionals with a broad view of the health/disease process that balances prevention and cure is reinforced, performing actions such as participating in the identification of Brazilian population problems under the responsibility of the health service and working in both multidisciplinary and intersectoral teams.

The reproduction of the biomedical model was also observed in USFs, indicating that practice seems to be more linked to the professional's training profile than to the type of service in which they work. In the dental profession, there are certain structural characteristics that give Oral Health its particularities, but make it difficult to practice in the public sector, such as the need to use hard technologies (equipment). This structural dependence conditions some resistance to changing the biomedical model, which is strongly supported by university training, the dental equipment and supplies industry and also by the social imaginary of the DS as a liberal professional working in a private clinic. It is therefore necessary to tackle the debate on oral health practices in order to build an expanded model of care and ensure that the population itself, which is used to consuming procedures in health services, is supported by adequate public policies to value health promotion (AQUILANTE & ACIOLE, 2015).

For the authors, the integrality of the health system refers to the articulation of the different levels of care, i.e. basic, specialized/secondary or hospital/tertiary, in such a way as to allow users to move through the system and have their health needs met, regardless of how or where they access it. Despite the progress made, the pyramid model in which PHC is placed as the obligatory gateway predominates. On the other hand, the issue of integrating services is one of the most serious impediments to comprehensive health care, since comprehensive actions are restricted to the USF under the principles of registration and linkage.

When actions at other levels of complexity are required, the system is vulnerable because it does not respond satisfactorily to the user's needs. There are established protocols regarding the scope of procedures at each level of care, which are still being adopted by professionals. When the RCR process is analyzed, it is clear that it is limited to bureaucratic issues and that each level of care leads the user to the services of another level.

According to the authors, faced with this situation, it is necessary to build a mechanism that really constitutes a shared production of care, since the specialties of prosthetics, periodontics and endodontics are the ones with the greatest repressed demands, with the latter having a waiting list that can reach more than two years, which compromises the continuity of care at the secondary and tertiary levels and leaves users in a situation of greater vulnerability to future mutilating treatments.

For Aquilante and Aciole (2015), it is true that scheduling has improved the population's access to oral health services since its inclusion in the ESF, although this access is largely restricted to the primary level of care. As a result, there is often inadequate referral to secondary and tertiary levels due to the lack of specialized services, which ends up generating excessive repressed demand. As a result, the comprehensive care provided to the registered population is not exercised by the DCs and, as a result, families do not have their needs and expectations met.

5   Methodological Procedures

5.1 Characterization of the study

According to the characteristics of this study and in order to answer its objectives, we opted for descriptive and exploratory research, with a qualitative approach, carried out in the form of a case study. According to Costa and Costa (2012), descriptive research describes and interprets a particular phenomenon, without interfering or modifying the reality studied.

According to Bauer and Gaskell (2008), descriptive research aims to describe the characteristics of a population, phenomenon or experience. At the end of a descriptive study, a lot of information is gathered and analyzed about the subject. The main contribution of this type of research is to provide new insights into an already known reality. Thus, it is a very specific type of research, as it consists of the in-depth and exhaustive study of a single object or a few objects (particular case), as it strongly depends on the context of the object to be studied and its results cannot be generalized.

According to Denzin and Lincoln (2000) exploratory research is carried out in areas and on issues where there is little or practically no accumulated or systematized knowledge, while Bauer and Gaskell (2008) state that descriptive and exploratory research is the most used by social researchers because they are always concerned with practical action.

The qualitative approach was defined for this study because it seeks to understand or give meaning to the behaviors or phenomena observed, without requiring a representative sample. In addition, this type of approach allows for communication with the research subjects and signals an intense collection of information, and the data collected can be represented verbally and with the possibility of numerical data. This type of approach takes into account more particular understandings, perceptions or psychic representations and therefore has an epistemological character since it takes into account personal considerations (COSTA & COSTA, 2012).

Conducting this research in the form of a case study allowed for an in-depth and detailed study of the case, since it was limited to three units, two of which were primary care and one secondary (COSTA & COSTA, 2012; DENZIN & LINCOLN, 2000).

5.2 Study scenario

The setting, according to Costa and Costa (2012), refers to the place where the research will be carried out and the justification for this choice. The study was carried out on Ilha do Governador, a neighborhood located in the North Zone of the municipality of Rio de Janeiro, in the mixed or "B" type primary care units, which bring together employees hired by the OS: Centro Municipal de Saù (CMS) Necker Pinto, in the Zumbi sub-borough; CMS Madre Teresa de Calcutà, in the Bancàrios sub-borough; and in the secondary care unit, the CEO, located in the Newton Alves Cardozo Polyclinic (PNAC). By studying these units, it was possible to analyze the practices involved in the articulation process established between these basic units and the CEO, in order to guarantee access to specialties to ensure continuity of care.

The two Municipal Health Centers (Centros Municipais de Saù - CMS) were selected for the study because they are the main primary care units in the neighborhood, with the largest catchment areas, which justifies the greater flow of RCR between primary and secondary care.

The study units are part of Program Area 3.1 (PA 3.1), which covers the neighborhoods of Bonsucesso to Jardim América, including Ilha do Governador, all located in the North Zone of the city. The health units cover Complexo do Alemao, Complexo da Maré, Complexo da Penha, Parque Royal, Dendê, Morro do Barbante, Vigàrio Geral and Parada de Lucas. In the last five years, there have been 131 family health teams in the 26 units of AP 3.1. There are 52 ESB teams and 14 Nùcleo de Apoio à Saùde da Familia teams. Planning Area 3.1 is divided into administrative regions and neighborhoods (IDEM).

Ilha do Governador corresponds to the XX Administrative Region. According to the 2010 IBGE Census, its total population was 212,547. This neighborhood is made up of six primary care units, four CMS and two Family Clinics (CF), which are: CMS Madre Teresa de Calcutà; CF Assis Valente; CF Maria Sebastiana de Oliveira; CMS Parque Royal; CMS Necker Pinto and CMS Paulino Werneck, as well as a secondary care unit, which is the Policlinica Newton Alves Cardoso. It also has an Emergency Care Unit (UPA) and two hospitals: the Evandro Freire Municipal Hospital (with 24-hour emergency care for highly complex cases) and the Nossa Senhora do Loreto Hospital (specializing in child care for cleft lip cases) (OTICS RIO, n.d.).

The Maria Sebastiana de Oliveira Health Center is located in the Moneró neighborhood. It has a type A care model and consists of six FH teams and two ESB teams. Its geographical catchment area is made up of a population of 27,000 inhabitants, with 18,891 people registered. This area covers the communities of Praia da Rosa, Morro do Dendê and Moneró (RIO DE JANEIRO, 2015c).

The Assis Valente FC, located in Galeao, has six FH teams and three ESB teams, benefiting approximately 24,000 residents of the Vila Joaniza and Barbante communities (OTICS RIO, n.d.).

The Paulino Werneck MHC, formerly the hospital of the same name, is located in Cacuia and is made up of three FH teams and two ESB teams; its catchment area is the Cacuia neighborhood (OTICS RIO, n.d.).

The Parque Royal MHC is located in the Portuguesa sub-borough and its catchment area is the same sub-borough located in the Ilha do Governador neighborhood - the Parque Royal Community. As for the registered population of this community, there is a total of 5,794 citizens, while the census carried out in 2010 by the IBGE shows that the Parque Royal community has 6,360 citizens; the unit has two FH teams (RIO DE JANEIRO, 2015b).

The CMS Necker Pinto, located in the neighborhood of Zumbi/Ilha do Governador, is primarily responsible for the neighborhoods of Zumbi, Praia da Bandeira, Ribeira, Pitangueiras, Nossa Senhora das Graças, Colònia Z10 and the surrounding area. The unit used to be classified as an ABS "C" model, *since* it didn't have an ESF. Today, however, after undergoing structural renovations to adapt and transform it, it is classified as a mixed unit, type "B", as it incorporates two FH teams and an ESB (CMS NECKER PINTO, undated).

The CMS Madre Teresa de Calcutà, located in Bairro dos Bancàrios/Ilha do Governador, is primarily responsible for the Bancàrios neighborhood, which "is situated 'at the foot' of Morro do INPS, surrounded by other communities such as: Bela Vista das Pixunas, Araras, Zaquias Jorge and Joao Telles de Menezes". Most of the clients served live in the Bancàrios neighborhood, followed by residents of Freguesia (including Bananal), Tauà (including Dendè), Moneró (part) and Cocotà. These areas are not currently fully covered by the ESF, and are the responsibility of the Unit through outpatient care. According to the Internal Regulations, the Unit has 43.86% coverage by the ESF, including the Bancàrios and Freguesia neighborhoods. The total population, according to the 2010 IBGE Census, is 72,869. The unit has four FHS teams and two ESBs (RIO DE JANEIRO, 2015a, s/p).

The Cadernos de Estatisticas e Mapas da Atença Primària em Saù of the municipality of Rio de Janeiro (CEMAPS RJ, 2013) establish that the units that develop PHC actions in the municipality of Rio de Janeiro are the CMS and the CF, classified as type A units where there are only FH teams and type B units where these teams coexist with other professionals from the unit (RIO DE JANEIRO, 2013).

The mission of the Oral Health Coordination, under the supervision and control of the Primary Care Superintendence, is to develop actions that promote comprehensive oral health care for the population of Rio de Janeiro, reversing epidemiological indicators and guaranteeing access to services. The work is based on an expanded concept of health and a systemic view of oral health, taking into account health indicators and the territory where these actions will be implemented. The Oral Health Program (PSB) is responsible for a network of dental services organized in a regionalized and hierarchical manner, offered in UBS, medium and high-complexity units and urgent/emergency care. The teams made up of specialized professionals include CDs, TSBs, ASBs and dental technicians (TPDs) (RIO DE JANEIRO, 2013).

According to the same reference, as a complement to primary care, the DSCs offer care in the areas of endodontics; specialized periodontics; minor oral surgery; stomatology; care for patients with special needs; preventive and interceptive orthodontics; and total and partial resin prostheses. To get specialized care, the user must go to the UBS of reference in their territory, which will carry out the initial assessment, the necessary basic treatment (educational, health promotion, preventive, restorative and surgical), as well as assessing the individual need for specialized treatment. If there is such a need, the patient will preferably be referred to the CEO in their area via the SISREG for vacancies, who will then inform them of the day, time and place of their specialist appointment.

It is worth noting that the PNAC CEO does not offer orthodontic or dental prosthesis services. It also provides care for patients with temporomandibular disorders (TMD).

5.3 Sampling

Sampling, understood as the process of obtaining the sample, was non-probabilistic, i.e. the selection of the sample "depends, at least in part, on the judgment of the researcher" and intentional, since the researcher used his judgment to select members of the population capable of providing information relevant to the study (COSTA & COSTA, 2012, p. 44).

5.4 Research Subjects

The research participants were the professionals involved in the RCR processes in Oral Health: DCs from the basic health units (CMS Necker Pinto and CMS Madre Tereza de Calcutà) and the CEO (Policlinica Newton Alves Cardoso); the professionals who are operationalizing the system's regulation process in these units and also the Oral Health coordinator in AP 3.1.

The study population consisted of three DCs from the Necker Pinto MHC, four DCs from the Madre Tereza de Calcutà MHC and seven DCs from the CEO, including a periodontist, an endodontist, a stomatologist, two specialists in temporomandibular dysfunction and orofacial pain, an oral and maxillofacial surgeon and an ESB DC. The sample size was therefore pre-established.

5.5 Data collection

In this study, the instrument selected for primary data collection was an individual interview, using a semi-structured script indicated, according to Costa and Costa (2012), to reach a small number of people, containing open and closed questions, and applied to the research subjects.

Through this instrument, we sought to understand and analyze whether there was integration between primary care and the secondary level (CEO), thus contemplating the implicit meaning of integrality, in an attempt to give greater objectivity to the discussion and reflection of the phenomena subordinated to the concept of integral health offered to SUS users.

The advantage of this instrument was that it allowed interaction with the interviewee, establishing a relationship of trust, as well as giving them the chance to talk about the topic in question without being tied to the question asked, but at the same time keeping them engaged.

focused on the theme in which the study's objectives were being sought. This allowed us to deepen our analysis of the subject, as well as allowing professionals to express themselves freely about the study's problem.

The interviewees did not give their consent for the interviews to be recorded, due to the fact that the professionals were overworked and were experiencing a huge increase in the number of patients as a result of the expanded access provided by the implementation of the ESF. Therefore, due to their refusal, the answers were recorded during the interviews, making the necessary records.

In this way, the meanings of the words were interpreted based on deduction, inference and reasoning. According to Costa and Costa (2012), this effort to interpret reasoning, rigorous in its objectivity and proficient in its subjectivity, is proof of the eagerness to perceive the hidden and the unsaid in the discourses obtained through the questionnaires.

In addition, so that the script could be improved in terms of the questions asked and the interviewer's attitude, a pilot test was carried out with another dentist from the oral health care network.

5.6 Data analysis

It can be said that the period of data analysis comprises the time following the collection of data and its consolidation.

Data analysis in this study was carried out in accordance with Bardin (2006), in terms of content analysis. She states that this tool consists of a set of techniques for analyzing communications and uses systematic and objective procedures to describe the content of messages, overcoming uncertainties and enriching the reading of the data collected. In order to achieve this goal, it is necessary to thoroughly read the statements collected through the interviews and coding procedures (PAB: primary care professionals; PCEO: CEO professionals; and PSIS: professionals who operate SISREG), categorization and subcategorization in order to achieve the research objectives.

As Chizzotti (2006, p. 98) states: "The aim of content analysis is to critically understand the meaning of communications, their manifest or latent content, their explicit or hidden meanings". Among communications, Bauer and Gaskell (2008) indicate that written textual materials are the most traditional in this type of analysis, and can be manipulated by the researcher in the search for answers to the research questions.

With a similar approach, Flick (2009, p. 291) states that content analysis "is one of the classic procedures for analyzing textual material, regardless of the origin of this material". Most of the time, there are various forms of documentation of the material collected, consisting of textual material, such as field notes, research diaries, documentation sheets, transcriptions, etc. However, the material can also be documented through photos, films, audios and so on, as all forms of documentation are relevant to the research process, enabling a proper analysis.

According to Vergara (2005), since content analysis is a technique that works on the data collected with the aim of identifying what is being said about a given topic, there is a need to decode what is being communicated. In order to decode the documents, the researcher can use various procedures, seeking to identify the most appropriate for the material to be analyzed, such as "lexical analysis, category analysis, enunciation analysis, connotation analysis" (CHIZZOTTI, 2006, p. 98).

For Minayo (2001, p. 74), content analysis is "understood much more as a set of techniques". For the author, it is the analysis of information about human behavior, allowing for a wide range of applications and has two functions: verification of hypotheses and/or questions and discovery of what lies behind the manifested contents. The process of data analysis itself involves several stages in order to give meaning to the data collected.

The study followed the stages of the technique, according to Bardin (2006), who organizes them into three phases: 1) Pre-analysis; 2) Exploration of the material; and 3) Treatment of the results, inference and interpretation.

The first phase, pre-analysis, is when the material to be analyzed is organized in order to make it operational, systematizing the initial ideas. For this research, specifically, the following organization was followed: 1) Floating reading, which is the establishment of contact with the data collection documents, a moment in which one begins to get to know the text; and 2) Choice of speeches, which consists of demarcating what will be analyzed.

The second phase involved analytical description, which refers to the *corpus* (any textual material collected) subjected to an in-depth study guided by the objects and the theoretical foundation.

The third phase concerns the treatment of the results, inference, discussion and interpretation. This stage is for processing the results, condensing and highlighting the information for analysis, culminating in inferential interpretations. This is the time for intuition, reflective and critical analysis. In view of the different phases proposed for content analysis, the dimensions of coding and categorization that enable and facilitate interpretations and inferences are highlighted, as the author herself did.

Flick (2009, p. 292-93) outlines the following steps for content analysis: "Synthesis of content analysis, by omitting statements and explanatory content analysis, by clarifying diffuse, ambiguous or contradictory passages", as well as "structuring content analysis, by structuring the formal level of the content".

The phases are therefore called "pre-analysis, analytical description and inferential interpretation, drawing attention to a fact". It is not possible for the researcher to focus exclusively on the manifest content of the documents, as they must deepen their analysis, trying to uncover the latent content they contain. Researchers who focus only on the manifest content of documents certainly belong to the positivist line (TRIVINOS, 1987, p. 162).

According to Campos (2004), categories can be aprioristic or non-aprioristic and he adds:

[...] we can characterize categories as large statements that encompass a variable number of themes, according to their degree of intimacy or proximity, and that can, through their analysis, express important meanings and elaborations that meet the objectives of the study and create new knowledge, providing a differentiated view of the proposed themes (p. 614).

In aprioristicas, the researcher, according to previous experience or interests, establishes pre-defined, wide-ranging categories, including subcategories that emerge from the text. It allows the researcher to directly classify their units of analysis within these categories and, from there, diversify them into subcategories. In the case of non-aprioristic categorization, these emerge entirely from the context, based on the answers given by the research subjects during the interviews, which requires the researcher to go back and forth between the material analyzed and the underlying theories, as well as not losing sight of the research objectives. The author reports that there are no magic formulas for categorization. "In general, the researcher follows his own path based on his theoretical knowledge, guided by his competence, sensitivity, intuition and experience." (p. 614).

This study used a priori categories or pre-categories related to the objectives of the research, to which the interview scripts (attached) were directed in accordance with what was recommended by Campos (2004). In this way, the data analyzed was organized into the respective **categories**, which are intrinsically linked to the Continuity of Care axis:

1) Offering oral health services;

2) Reference and appointment;

3) Counter-referral;

4) Strengths and weaknesses; and

5) Professionals' perception.

We believe that the data selected met the objectives of the research and addressed the central question of how the link between primary care and the DSC at the site investigated is processed in order to guarantee continuity of care. In addition, during the process of analyzing the data, some subcategories emerged which had not previously been foreseen.

During the analysis of the category "supply of oral health services", four subcategories had to be created in order to emphasize important aspects found when reading the data: supply/demand ratio, statistical records, institutional support and logistics. Similarly, in the "referral and scheduling" category, two subcategories emerged: training and continuing education and communication and information resources.

5.7 Ethical aspects

With regard to ethical aspects, and in accordance with Resolution 466/12 of the National Health Council, the project was submitted to the Research Ethics Committee of the municipality of Rio de Janeiro, as three units were studied in its territory. In addition, the participants received an Informed Consent Form (ICF), a model of which is available in the "Appendix".

6 Results and Discussion

6.1 Profile of the interviewees

- **Sex**

Of the seven UBS professionals, six (85.7%) were female and one (14.2%) male. Of the seven CEO professionals interviewed, four (57%) were female and three (43%) male. The four professionals who operate SISREG, two DCs, a THD and an administrative assistant, are all female. This reflects the predominance of women in dentistry and in the health job market.

Forty years ago, the profession could have been considered masculine, as around 90% of professionals were men. The change in this profile began to be observed from the end of the 1990s, in line with the increased education of women in the country. The greater presence of women is also seen in other areas of health. Women's choice of this career also has peculiar reasons, "such as the possibility of a flexible working day, some degree of mobility, with the possibility of moving to start a family, and the relative social prestige of the profession" (JORNAL ODONTO, 2010, s/p).

According to the Brazilian Dental Association (ABO), women are the majority in the profession. They represent around 52% in 25 of Brazil's 27 states, except for Santa Catarina and Acre. The data comes from the survey "Current Profile and Trends of the Brazilian Dental Surgeon", carried out by the Faculty of Dentistry of the University of São Paulo, in partnership with the Ministry of Health and the Pan American Health Organization, with the support of the ABO. Dentistry confirms a worldwide trend: according to data from the Federal Council of Dentistry (CFO), women represent almost 64% of registered professionals in the country, while men still prevail only in the over 56 age group (NAVARRO, 2012).

- **Age group**

The average age of PHC interviewees is 37.7 years. Statutory primary care professionals have an average age of 45.5 years, while ESB professionals have an average age of 27.3 years.

In the case of the CEO interviewees, this average is 42.7 years. The permanent professionals have an average age of 45.8 years, while the CD who makes up the ESB is only 24 years old. Among the interviewees who operate SISREG, the average age is 39.25, with the youngest professional being 27 and the oldest 52.

Generally speaking, it can be seen that permanent staff are older than those hired by the OSS. This can be related to the greater maturity acquired by these professionals and their greater experience in the work they do: "It can't be denied that more mature people still have a lot to contribute. They have accumulated a lot of experience and still have vitality" (COSTA, 2007, s/p).

- **Professional relationship**

The PHC units studied are of the "mixed or B" type, since they underwent structural reforms to adapt and transform them by incorporating ESF and ESB (CMS NECKER PINTO, n/d and RIO DE JANEIRO, 2015a, s/p).

The graph below shows the distribution of UABs in AP 3.1, according to a survey carried out by the Municipality of Rio de Janeiro's Municipal Health Department.

Graph 1 - Distribution of BA units by type (A, B and C) in PA 3.1.

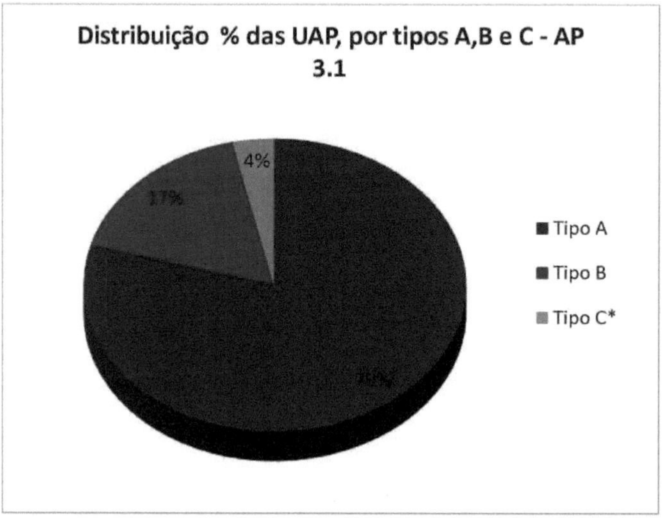

Source: SB coordination of the Municipal Health Department of Rio de Janeiro (2017).

Thus, the type B units bring together statutory (permanent) professionals who were already working in the unit before the ESF was set up and professionals who were hired by the Health Organizations (OS) to make up the ESB.

With regard to the professional relationship of primary care DSs, the survey found that the three professionals (42.8%) who make up the ESB were hired temporarily under the Consolidation of Labor Laws (CLT), while the four professionals (57.2%) who already belonged to the units are statutory (permanent).

As for the CEO's seven DCs, the survey found that there is only one professional (14.3%) who makes up the ESB, who was hired temporarily under the Consolidated Labor Laws (CLT), while the other six (85.7%), who already belonged to the unit, are statutory (permanent).

With regard to the professionals who operate SISREG, the two dental hygienists who make up the

ESB and the administrative professional who works at the NIR (Núcleo Interno de Regulaçao) at the Madre Tereza de Calcutà MHC were hired temporarily under the CLT regime, while the THD (Dental Hygiene Technician) at the Necker Pinto MHC is a statutory employee.

Within the legal framework of health policy, the LOS and Law No. 8.142/90, programs must be based on parameters of access, reception, linkage and resolubility, in order to provide good care for users (BRASIL, 2011).

According to Giovanella and Mendonça (2008), care directed at populations in defined territories, assuming health responsibility for them and considering the local dynamics of these populations, should be guided by the principles of universality, accessibility, coordination and continuity of care, establishment of a link, humanization, social participation, among others.

According to Oliveira and Pereira (2013), the organization of primary health care services, through the ESF, prioritizes actions to promote, protect and recover comprehensive health, continuously contemplating practices and services that go beyond medical care and are based on the needs of the population, which are apprehended from the establishment of bonds between users and professionals.

This raises questions about the possibility of hiring the professionals who make up the ESB through the OSS, since it is not an actual hiring, but rather the establishment of a temporary employment relationship for the professionals, which could be detrimental to the consolidation of integrality and continuity of care.

According to the research carried out by Serra and Rodrigues (2010), with regard to human resources, it was observed that there are professionals with temporary functional contracts, which causes damage to integrality.

- **Workload**

With regard to the workload in the institution, the survey found that the professionals who make up the ESB work a full 40-hour week, while the statutory professionals, who already belonged to the basic units, work a 24-hour week, with the exception of the professionals who hold management positions, who work a 40-hour week.

With regard to the professionals who operate SISREG, the ESB DCs and the administrative professional at the Madre Tereza de Calcutà MHC work a full 40-hour week, as does the THD (statutory) at the Necker Pinto MHC.

- **Professional training**

With regard to the training of the professionals, there are different situations. At CMS Necker Pinto, both the patients referred by the ESB and the patients referred by the statutory DCs are entered into SISREG by the unit's THD. At CMS Madre Tereza de Calcutta, there are two different situations: the ESB patients are referred by the DCs themselves and the patients of the statutory DCs are referred by an administrative employee of the NIR.

CAP 3.1 has its own NIR which develops strategic actions aimed at organizing the regulation of consultations, exams and hospitalizations in AP 3.1. The units are instructed to set up their own Internal Regulation Units, made up of professionals trained in regulation in SISREG (Regulation System) by the Municipal Regulation Center.

In this context, it should be emphasized that dental professionals, such as the DCs and THDs themselves, find it easier to identify nomenclature specific to the field of dentistry, unlike the NIR's administrative assistant, who, despite being trained to operate the system, does not have specific knowledge related to dentistry. This situation can lead to referral errors and consequently harm to the patient.

- **Time since graduation**

With regard to length of training, permanent primary care professionals have an average of 21.5 years of training, while those who make up the ESB have an average of five years.

As for the CEO professionals, the permanent ones have an average of 23.6 years of training, while the ESB professionals have only two years.

In this context, it can be seen that statutory DCs have a longer period of training, which means they have more professional experience than those hired by the OS, who make up the ESB.

With regard to the length of time the professionals who operate SISREG have been trained, the THD has eight years, the DCs, five and eight years and the administrative assistant, 15 years.

- **Time working for SUS**

With regard to the length of time they have been working in the Unified Health System (SUS), permanent primary care professionals have an average of 19.75 years, while ESB DCs have been working in the SUS for an average of 1.7 years. Effective DSC professionals have an average age of 16.3 years and the ESB CD has only been working in the SUS for one year.

As for the professionals who operate SISREG, the THD is eight years old, one CD is only eight months old and the other is four years old, while the NIR administrative employee is one year old.

In this respect, it can be seen that permanent professionals have been working in the SUS for a longer period of time, which helps them to establish a relationship, unlike the professionals recently hired by the OS, who have temporary employment contracts, which is a negative aspect when it comes to establishing a relationship with the population.

• **Professional training**

The survey found that four PHC interviewees (57.14%) had received training to carry out their role in PHC, while three (42.85%) reported not having been trained. Five (71.4%) interviewees from the DSC had not received any training to carry out their work in the DSC and only two DCs (28.6%) reported having been trained. With regard to the professionals who operate SISREG, two (50%) said they had been trained and two (50%) said they had not.

Thus, with regard to human resources, professionals without appropriate training, lack of training for the job and precarious permanent education jeopardize integrality (SERRA & RODRIGUES, 2010).

In addition, according to Scheffer *et al* (2010), the care that is considered ideal should be provided in services of excellence by professionals who combine training, updating and professional experience.

The tables below summarize the profile of the professionals interviewed. It is worth noting that acronyms or codes have been adopted for each interviewee in order to preserve confidentiality (PAB: primary care professional, PCEO: CEO professional and PSIS: professional who operates SISREG):

Chart 1 - Profile of PC professionals interviewed.

ATTRIBUTES	PABI	PAB2	PAB3	PAB4	PAB5	PAB6	PAB7
SEX	F	F	F	F	M	F	F
AGE	38 YEARS	44 YEARS	27 YEARS	32 YEARS	54 YEARS	46 YEARS	23 YEARS
VINCULO	EFFECTIVE	EFFECTIVE	CLT	CLT	EFFECTIVE	EFFECTIVE	CLT
TRAINING TIME	16 YEARS	22 YEARS	6 YEARS	7 YEARS	24 YEARS	24 YEARS	2 YEARS
SUS TIME	14 YEARS	21 YEARS	4 YEARS	8 MONTHS	22 YEARS	22 YEARS	6 MONTHS
TRAINING	NO	NO	YES	NO	YES	YES	YES

Source: own elaboration using survey data.

Chart 2 - Profile of the CEO professionals interviewed.

ATTRIBUTES	PCEO1	PCEO2	PCEO3	PCEO4	PCEO5	PCEO6	PCEO7
SEX	F	F	M	F	M	F	M
AGE	49 YEARS	40 YEARS	47 YEARS	52 YEARS	44 YEARS	43 YEARS	24 YEARS
VINCULO	EFFECTIVE	EFFECTIVE	EFFECTIVE	EFFECTIVE	EFFECTIVE	EFFECTIVE	CLT
TRAINING TIME	27 YEARS	17 YEARS	24 YEARS	30 YEARS	22 YEARS	22 YEARS	2 YEARS
SUS TIME	20 YEARS	14 YEARS	13 YEARS	14 YEARS	22 YEARS	15 YEARS	1 YEAR
TRAINING	NO	YES	NO	NO	NO	NO	YES

Source: own elaboration using survey data.

Chart 3 - Profile of the professionals interviewed who operate SISREG.

ATTRIBUTES	PSIS1	PSIS 2	PSIS 3	PSIS 4
SEX	F	F	F	F
AGE	46 YEARS	27 YEARS	32 YEARS	52 YEARS
VíNCULO	EFFECTIVE	CLT	CLT	CLT
TRAINING TIME	8 YEARS	5 YEARS	7 YEARS	15 YEARS
SUS TIME	8 YEARS	4 YEARS	8 MONTHS	1 YEAR
TRAINING	YES	NO	YES	NO

Source: own elaboration using survey data.

- **Oral Health Coordination Profile**

During the research, the Oral Health Coordinator of AP 3.1 was represented by the Oral Health Advisor of CAP 3.1, the dental surgeon Dr. Patricia Coelho de Oliveira e Silva Almeida, who readily agreed to take part in the research, including providing data that corroborated the study. She is 23 years old, has a permanent professional contract, has worked in the SUS for 20 years and has held her current position for two years.

6.2 Thematic Axis and Categories of Analysis

In accordance with the methodological design adopted, we believe that the principle of comprehensiveness, understood in this work as continuity of care, runs throughout the analysis of the research results, constituting the only thematic axis. Thus, each a priori category created from this broad axis absorbed the results identified with the proposed objectives and, in this way, were analyzed and discussed in order to provide concrete elements to answer them.

The table below shows the thematic axis, which refers to comprehensiveness in the sense of continuity of care, and its respective categories of analysis:

Chart 4 - Thematic axis and categories of analysis.

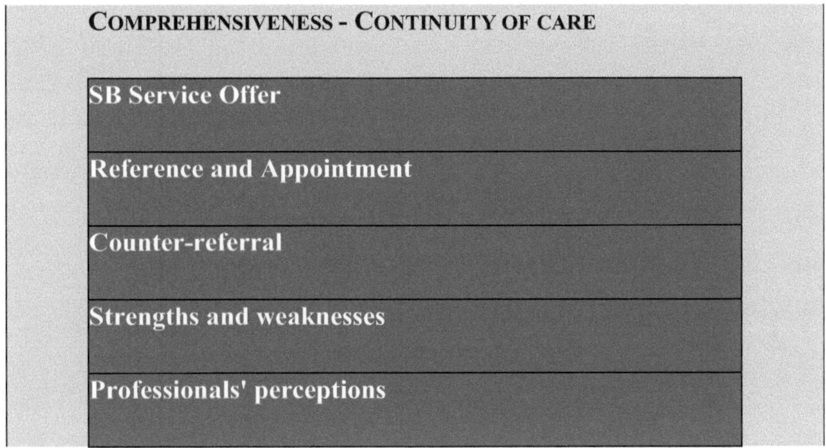

COMPREHENSIVENESS - CONTINUITY OF CARE

Source: own elaboration based on the theoretical foundation.

Category: Buccal Health services

In this category, two fundamental aspects were highlighted for analysis and discussion: primary and secondary care services and the complementary exams needed for oral health diagnosis and treatment. In order to deepen and build knowledge about the object, the following subcategories were created: supply/demand relationship, statistical record, institutional support, logistics.

- Specialized Services

The Basic Health Units (UBS) carry out basic dental procedures, such as: oral hygiene instruction, caries removal and restoration, basic periodontal therapy (prophylaxis and supra-gingival scraping), simple tooth extraction, health promotion, among others (RIO DE JANEIRO, 2011).

"We do basic periodontal therapy, restorations, extractions and health promotion" (PAB1).

"PHC is the main axis of the HCN, and is responsible for the whole process of coordinating care, facilitating integration between the points of the network. We carry out examinations, chairside care, such as scraping, direct restorations, access and exodontia, we also carry out oral health promotion groups, among others provided for by PHC" (PAB3).

Thus, according to the Ministry of Health, primary care is responsible for providing oral health care until all therapeutic possibilities have been exhausted at primary level. Then, when the possibility of treatment at this level of care is exceeded and more complex dental procedures are required, the patient is referred to the CEO (BRASIL, 2004b).

"treatments that are not available in primary care will be carried out at the CEO" (PAB2).

On Ilha do Governador, the CEO works at the PNAC (Newton Alves Cardoso Polyclinic) and, according to the survey, provides oral health care in the following specialties: Periodontics, Minor Oral Surgery, Endodontics, Patients with Special Needs, Stomatology and TMD (Temporomandibular Disorder).

According to the CEO, specialized consultations are offered to primary care patients on a weekly basis, as follows:

Chart 5 - Specialized consultations offered weekly by the CEO to patients at AB.

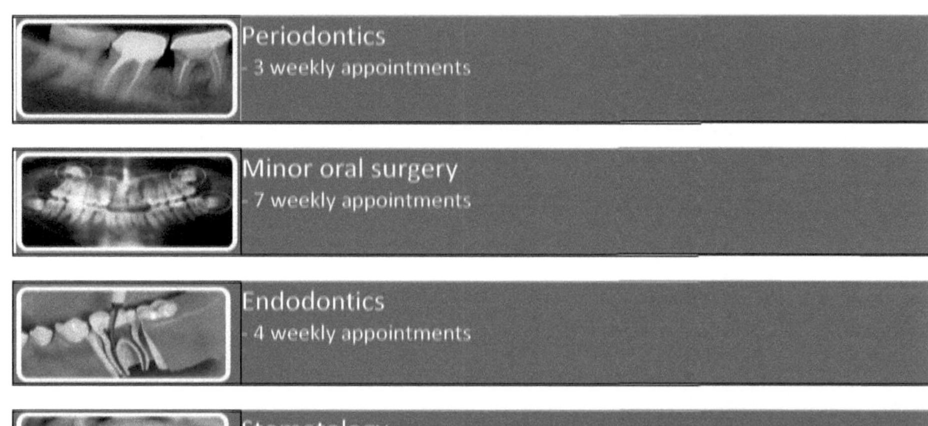

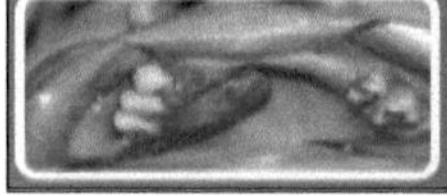

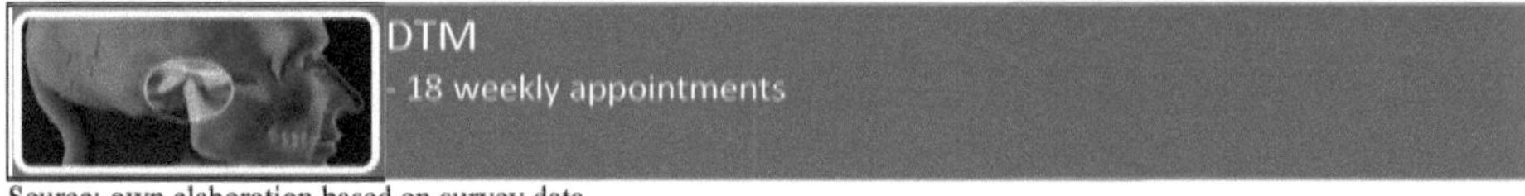

Source: own elaboration based on survey data.

The referral of the patient from the UBS to the CEO is done via the regulation system (SISREG), which regulates the vacancies offered to the PHC. Thus, the CEO offers the vacancy in the specialty, defining the date and time of the consultation, the regulation center, which communicates the UBS, which in turn contacts the patient to make the appointment, as analyzed in the following statements:

"the primary care unit refers the patient to the CEO, through SISREG, which regulates the vacancies... the CEO makes the vacancies available weekly to the regulation center, which will notify the unit that referred the patient to a certain specialty" (PCEO1).

"The dentist refers the patient to a specialty, such as endodontics, surgery, stomatology, etc. Then I enter the request or need into SISREG... Then the regulation center notifies us when a vacancy arises at the CEO for that specialty, giving the day and time of the appointment, and we call to tell the patient about the appointment at the CEO" (PSIS1).

Thus, in everyday practice, users who are seen in primary care, after all therapeutic possibilities have been exhausted, are referred to specialized care, which is carried out at the CEO. This process is regulated through a computerized system which, according to the Ministry of Health, aims to guarantee access to exams, specialist consultations and hospitalizations at the most complex levels by referring patients (BRASIL, 2006b).

When asked about the specialties with the highest number of referrals to the DSC, the PHC and DSC professionals and the OH coordination itself highlighted endodontics first, minor oral surgery second and stomatology third.

Figure 1 - Specialties with the highest number of referrals to the CEO.

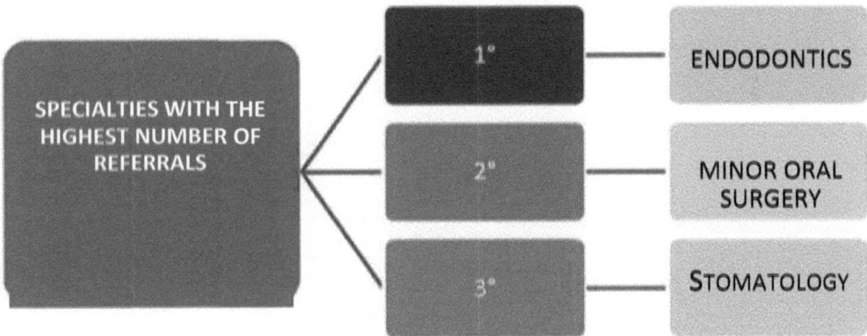

Source: own elaboration based on survey data.

Thus, it can be seen that for both primary care and CEO DCs, endodontics was considered the specialty with the highest number of referrals, i.e. the highest demand. This should be taken into account by the manager when planning the supply of services, avoiding the occurrence of waiting lines caused by the disproportion between supply and demand.

Pimentel *et al* (2010) observed, in a study on the referral of patients to medium and high complexity services, some difficulties both in the lack of agreements for certain municipal services and in the evident accumulated demand, especially for the specialty of endodontics. These authors state that if the needs of the local service are not resolved, there is no RCR scheme and the problems remain unsolved, as users cannot afford treatment in the private network. As a result, dentistry is unable to solve the oral problems of its population because of the huge demand that has built up.

In Rio de Janeiro, this task falls to the Computerized Regulation System (SISREG), which is also responsible for oral health appointments (BRASIL, 2006b). SISREG's objectives include:

According to Giovanella *et al* (2009), it is the concern of all managers to integrate the care network; in order to integrate primary care with medium complexity, the strategy used was to set up computerized regulation centers in order to control flows and optimize resources through sufficient supply, the establishment of clinical priorities and the monitoring of waiting lists.

For the authors, the system would also make it possible to monitor the user's journey, reducing the number of absentees, queues and waiting times, as well as making it possible to redistribute quotas between health centers, contract supply according to demand, analyze referrals and control agendas more impartially. It should be added that the effectiveness of integration is conditioned by supply, which is often not enough to meet the demand for specialized services, generating waiting lists.

According to the Health Coordination, the waiting lists are monitored and this problem is being tackled:

"through the management of lists by the head of the CEO and the periodic analysis of data relating to appointments, absenteeism..." (SB coordination).

Thus, according to the SB coordination, management actions have been taken with the aim of tackling the problem of pent-up demand and waiting lines, but what we see in practice is that these measures have not been enough to resolve this deficiency, which hinders the flow of dental care, harming the user of the system.

- Complementary tests for diagnosis and treatment

Complementary tests provide the information needed to diagnose an alteration or disease. The request for a complementary examination must take into account the data obtained through the anamnesis and physical examination, knowing exactly what is to be obtained and correctly understanding the value and limitations of the requested examination.

Radiographic imaging exams are commonly used in all specialties and are therefore frequently used in dentistry. These examinations are used to assess oral lesions, especially when they affect bone tissue, such as the maxilla and mandible, and lesions that affect tooth structure, such as caries. In certain situations, radiography will be conclusive, such as in the detection of foreign bodies, retained teeth, partial anodontia, root fractures and positional anomalies.

The radiographic examinations normally requested by the UBS are periapical and panoramic radiographs. Panoramic X-rays give a general idea of the teeth, facial bones and skull, without too much detail. However, when you want detailed information about just one tooth, for example, it is preferable to take a periapical radiograph, which shows images with greater precision and a wealth of detail (e.g. initial canals, root canal treatment, etc.) (w2.fop.unicamp.br/).

In the case of the PNAC CEO, there is a device for taking periapical radiographs, however:

"It hasn't been used because the unit's professionals aren't receiving the dangerousness bonus, as provided for in the legislation" (PSIS1).

Thus, when a periapical radiograph is needed to complement the diagnosis, a referral must be made via SISREG, and it is carried out in units outside the neighborhood of Ilha do Governador. This leads to users giving up because of the waiting time, the distance and the cost of travel, **and** opting to have these tests carried out at clinics or private practices in their own neighborhood.

"When you need an X-ray, I refer you through SISREG, which gives you a place at another CEO, off the island, and that's why most patients prefer to go to a private clinic, right here in the neighborhood, because it's cheaper and easier than leaving the island" (PSIS1).

It can be seen that the lack of availability of this test in the neighborhood unit, which means that patients have to travel to another CEO, further away, leads most patients to opt for the test in the private network, as it is faster, more practical and even less expensive. This situation has *already* been studied by authors such as Serra and Rodrigues (2010), who found that among the operational deficiencies that compromise the proper functioning of the RCR is the lack of planning, which in this case refers to a random spatial distribution of the units.

In the case of panoramic X-rays, the referral unit is the Nossa Senhora do Loreto Municipal Hospital, which specializes in treating children with cleft lip and is located in the same neighbourhood. However, in order to have this test carried out, the patient must also be referred via the Vacancy Regulation System, which most of the time leads the user to also opt for the private network.

"I make the referral via SISREG and the panoramic X-ray is taken at Loreto Hospital" (PSIS3).

"Here, patients always prefer to have a private scan, because it's a cheap test that patients can afford, and it's quicker, because you don't have to wait for a SISREG slot" (PSIS1).

This shows that although the network provides the exam at a hospital in the neighborhood, it is located in the Galeao region and is further away from the UABs studied and the CEO. Thus, the majority of patients opt to have the test done in the private network due to the distance and the delay in booking the test via SISREG, considering it to be faster and more practical, due to the limited supply of tests, as shown by Mapal:

Map 1: AP Units 3.1.

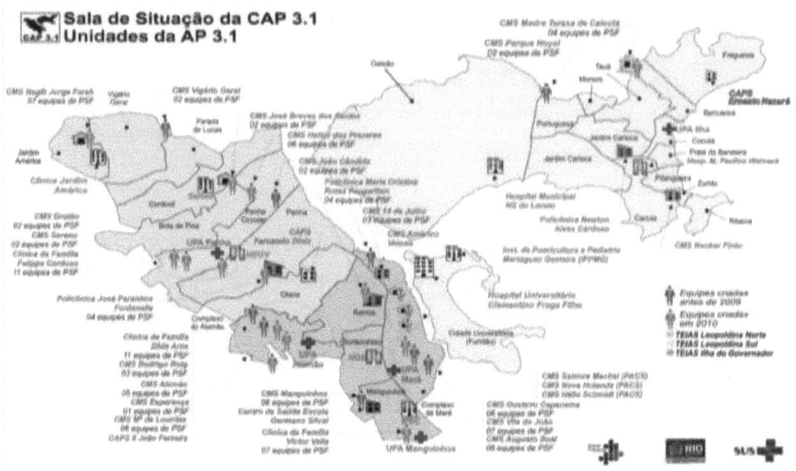

Source: Blog of the Health Coordination of Planning Area 3.1 (CAP 3.1). Available at: http://cap31.blogspot.com.br/2011/04/unidades-da-ap-31-versao-abril2011.html.

Serra and Rodrigues (2010) report that among the items that hinder patient access and the proper functioning of the RCR system are: "(1) limited supply of consultations and exams [...]; (3) poor organization of regulation activities" (p. 3,579).

The same authors report on the concept of comprehensiveness, provided for as a guideline by the Federal Constitution and as a principle by the LOS, which refers to the right of users to access the actions of the different levels of complexity, with defined and spatially organized flows in order to ensure continuity of care in units located close to the citizens. Thus, for them, the difficulty of access due to financial problems, such as the cost of tickets, hampers the effective functioning of the RCR. This refers to inadequate sizing in relation to demand, which also shows a lack of planning (SERRA E RODRIGUES, 2010).

Subcategory: supply/demand ratio

Regarding the availability of specialized consultations and exams to meet the needs of patients at the Primary Care Unit, three (42.8%) interviewees from the CEO reported that they did, three (42.8%) reported that they didn't and one (14.4%) reported that they didn't know.

Regarding the existence of sufficient services to meet the needs of primary care, the following statements were recorded:

"SISREG organizes the supply of vacancies, which depends on the availability of each professional" (PCEO6).

"Initially, vacancies are offered through SISREG on a weekly basis" (PCEO1).

It can be seen that vacancies are made available on a weekly basis, but the number of vacancies is offered according to the availability of existing professionals and not according to patient demand.

With regard to the number of professionals being sufficient, all (100%) of the professionals at the CEO were unanimous in saying that it was not:

"this is justified by the length of time the patient has to wait in line" (PCEO7).

"There has been an expansion of the ESF, but on the other hand there is a lack of incentive and resources for the CEO... because there is a lot of pent-up demand" (PCEO1).

"demand is high and there has been no possibility of prioritizing care yet" (PCEO4).

"With the expansion of primary care in the municipality, the increase in the population covered and the family clinics, our secondary care network has not received any specialized professionals, which would increase the supply of specialized vacancies... through a survey of SISREG reports and monitoring with the CEOs, we were able to justify to the local coordination the need to bring in some specialized professionals, such as periodontists,... for our CEOs" (SB coordination). to our CEOs" (SB coordination).

Thus, the statements reinforced that there has not been a sufficient number of professionals to meet the needs of the local population, which in turn has been growing as a result of the expansion of the ESF, which has increased the registered population. However, this expansion has not been carried out in the same proportion in secondary care, which has not increased the number of professionals, which has led to pent-up demand and a waiting list.

Graph 2 - Number of families registered in AP 3.1 - 2009 to October 2015.

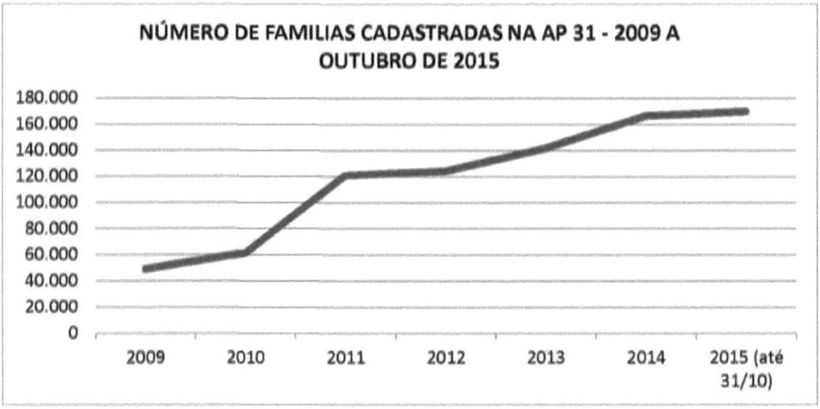

Source: SB coordination of the Municipal Health Department of Rio de Janeiro (2017).

Santos and Assis (2006) analyzed the practice of oral health and also found that it has been organized through individual and collective actions, built by a repressed demand, with fragmented care and the excessive valorization of technique and specialty whose axis is ordered by the medical-centered model, with limited resolubility, in a tense and conflicting relationship.

For Aquilante and Aciole (2015), the integrality of the health system refers to the articulation of the different levels of care, so that users can move through the system and have their health needs met. On the other hand, the integration of services is one of the most serious impediments to comprehensive health care, since comprehensive actions are restricted to the USF. When actions at other levels of complexity are required, the system is vulnerable, as it does not respond satisfactorily to the user's needs.

According to the authors, some specialties, such as endodontics, have the highest backlogs, with a waiting list that can reach more than two years, which compromises continuity of care and leaves users more vulnerable to future mutilating treatments.

According to the authors, scheduling has improved the population's access to oral health services since its inclusion in the ESF. However, there is often inadequate referral to secondary and tertiary levels due to the lack of specialized services, which ends up generating excessive repressed demand. As a result, the comprehensive care provided to the population is not exercised and, as a result, families do not have their needs and expectations met.

Subcategory: statistical recording

When asked if they keep any statistical records of the demand for their specialty, four (57.2%) CEO interviewees said no, while three (42.8%) said yes.

With regard to records for statistical control in order to gather data for management, the following statements were obtained:

"I control the discharges" (PCEO3).

"The record is made by writing off the consultations through their confirmation in SISREG... every specialist is obliged to return the patient on discharge from the specialty, with the counter-referral, putting their name in a book and the patient signs it. This is done at the PNAC CEO" (PCEO1).

It can be seen that DSC professionals have recorded the discharges of patients who were referred by the PC to the DSC after the specialized procedure was completed. This measure makes it possible to collect data that is important for action planning, but only takes into account cases that have been attended to, and does not take into account repressed demand.

According to Serra and Rodrigues (2010), who studied some of the operational deficiencies that hinder the smooth running of the RCR between PHC and the other levels of complexity, it became clear in that context that the management bodies do not have effective control over the secondary units due to the lack of planning, regulation and political appointment of the heads of these units. It is therefore essential for managers to be attentive to the use of resources for records, with the aim of collecting data that will corroborate the planning of actions and services.

According to Rodrigues and Santos (2011), information must always be available and up-to-date. In addition, the actions taken must be monitored and evaluated with a view to intervening and making corrections if necessary. However, the same authors also report that the SUS does not present itself as an effectively integrated system, because, in a large part of the country, there are deficiencies in the information, communication and logistics systems, as well as in the planning and control bodies.

Subcategory: institutional support

With regard to CEO professionals receiving institutional support to clarify doubts, two (28.5%) interviewees said no, while all the others (71.5%) said yes.

The SB coordinator said that the professionals are supported in relation to doubts and difficulties, and that this support is provided through email, phone calls to the SB advisory office and the group on social networks (*WhatsApp*).

In the research carried out by Serra and Rodrigues (2010), the lack of technical support for the teams was noted, which makes it difficult for professionals to make decisions and increases the number of referrals.

Subcategory: logistics

In this subcategory, two fundamental aspects were analyzed and discussed: maintenance of equipment and inputs.

- **Equipment maintenance**

Dentistry is a clinic that relies on the use of a wide range of equipment in order to carry out its activities. It is therefore considered an expensive service, due to the investment in technological resources, as well as the need for constant calibration and maintenance of this equipment.

In the dental profession, there are certain structuring characteristics that give Oral Health its particularities, but hinder its practice in the public sector, such as the need to use hard technologies (equipment). This structural dependence conditions some resistance to changing the biomedical model, which is strongly supported by university training, the dental equipment and supplies industry and also by the social imaginary of the DS as a liberal professional working in a private clinic (AQUILANTE AND ACIOLE, 2015).

When asked if the equipment in the PHC unit receives constant maintenance, the professionals were unanimous (100%) in saying that it does. The same question was asked of the DSC professionals and only two DCs (28.5%) said no, while the rest (71.5%) said yes. *The* SB coordinator said that *the* equipment used is regularly maintained and calibrated.

As for the frequency of this maintenance, the professionals said that it is carried out every two weeks to every month. However, it is worth noting that, despite the constant technical visits to maintain the equipment, there are still reports of problems.

"They receive maintenance frequently, but many problems arise despite this maintenance" (PCEO6).

The study carried out by Serra and Rodrigues (2010) **on** logistical support showed that poor maintenance and calibration of biomedical equipment leads to errors in diagnoses and improper prescriptions, with serious consequences for patients.

In addition, it is clear that faulty equipment makes it impossible to provide adequate patient care, or even prevents it from being provided at all, causing great damage to the guarantee of dental care for the user.

- **Inputs**

With regard to the lack of supplies for carrying out their activities, six (85.7%) of those interviewed from primary care replied that this does not occur in primary care and only one CD (14.3%) reported a lack of light-curing resin. Among the CEO professionals, only two (28.5%) of the interviewees said that it doesn't happen, while all the others (71.5%) said that it does.

With regard to the lack of inputs, the interviewees said:

"There's no plaque, no material for infiltration when necessary" (PCEO2).

"lack of acetate plate to make intraoral device" (PCEO4).

"lack of adequate suture thread, surgical field" (PCEO5).

"supplies are lacking in all specialties" (PCEO3).

"there are some occasional shortages" (PCEO1).

According to the SB coordinator, there is planning and stock control for the materials and supplies used in the services, but he also considered that there is a lack of materials, more modern equipment and supplies.

When asked about the average waiting time for the necessary materials, the professionals interviewed had this to say:

"the waiting time is about a month" (PCEO3).

"Previously, we received it every four months. Now, for about a year, we've been exchanging materials with other CEOs. So we're asking for emergency purchases through CAP 3.1" (PCEO1).

"for example, we've been waiting for the plaque since 2012" (PCEO2).

"from 4 to 6 months... the purchase depends on the processes carried out and authorized by the central level, through a bidding process" (SB coordination).

In addition to the use of equipment, dentistry has other structural peculiarities that also hinder its practice, such as the need to use dental supplies (AQUILANTE & ACIOLE, 2015).

These supplies are essential for carrying out the services, especially the specialized ones, performed at the CEO. The survey showed that the lack of supplies makes it difficult for professionals to carry out their activities, which consequently makes it impossible to guarantee the continuity of dental care.

Category: reference and scheduling

In this category, the research sought to analyze and discuss the criteria adopted by dental surgeons for referring users registered at the Zumbi and Bancàrios units to the secondary unit, as well as describing how scheduling for specialized oral health appointments works. It is worth noting that two subcategories emerged during the analysis of this category: training and continuing education and communication and information resources.

There is no informality in the structure of the units studied when it comes to referring patients. There are defined formal structures, through forms (ANNEX) containing some information that is necessary for the development of patient referrals from the PHC to the DSC, established with the oral health coordinator.

According to Silva (2009), the RCR is part of a "puzzle" that drives the rational use of levels of complexity and makes the SUS productive, undoing the knots that hinder the system, facilitating integrality in terms of user access and continuity of care.

It should also be noted that, according to Serra and Rodrigues (2010), the integration of health networks is guaranteed by an effective system of RCRs, which establishes the mutual referral of patients between the different levels of complexity of the services. In addition, with regard to clinical management, the authors found that the use of clinical protocols and referrals supported by clinical protocols and guidelines is fundamental.

With regard to referrals to the DSC being made after all clinical resources at the PHC have been exhausted, all the DCs interviewed from the PHC (100%) agreed. According to Campos *et al* (2010), PHC should be one of the main entry points to the health system; however, much more is expected of it than just the function of guaranteeing access to the system, such as the ability to solve around 80% of problems while the remaining cases would be referred, thus making up an articulated network of services that expands the capacity to solve patients' health problems in a comprehensive manner.

With regard to the use of some form for referring patients from primary care to the DSC, all (100%) were aware of it and confirmed its use. Pimentel *et al* (2010) report that, according to the Caderno da Atença Bàsica - Saùde Bucal, referrals should be made using RCR forms, accompanied or not by complementary exams and X-rays.

In such a way that at the UBS, when there is a need for specialized dentistry, after all the basic therapeutic possibilities have been exhausted, the patient is referred to the CEO at the Newton Alves Cardoso Polyclinic (PNAC), which serves all the UBS on Ilha do Governador. The PNAC, in turn, passes on vacancies for specialized services to the Central Regulation Office, which notifies the referral unit, which will book or schedule the patient's appointment.

The PNAC CEO is a reference for all the AB units on Ilha do Governador and has the following specialties: Periodontics, Endodontics, TMD, Minor Oral Surgery, Stomatology and Care for Patients with Special Needs.

The protocols recommended and adopted in practice by the units are those proposed by the Ministry of Health in accordance with Notebook 17 of the PHC Notebooks. The study identified some restrictions and observations contained in the specialty protocols, which should be followed by UBS dentists when referring their patients to the CEO specialties and which can be briefly described as follows:

Chart 6 - Restrictions and observations for referrals to endodontics, periodontics, minor oral surgery and patients with special needs.

endodontics		periodontics		minor oral surgery		patients with special needs	
	-Preferably permanent teeth; -Do not refer a tooth when there is a need for prosthetic treatment afterwards; - Remove all decayed tissue and make access; -Do not refer a 3rd molar; -Do not refer endodontic retreatment; - When possible, try capping; and - Adjust the oral environment before referring.		-Preparing the oral environment; - Preparing supra-gingival scraping; - Carefully assessing cases of tooth mobility; and - Controlling and monitoring the patient after discharge from the DSC should be done at the BHU.		-Avoid sending simple surgeries; - Avoid sending residual roots; -Send more complex surgeries such as extraction of wisdom teeth, serial extractions and subgingival roots that require osteotomy; - Prepare anamnesis of the patient to find out if they are fit to undergo the procedure; and -Suture removal will be carried out at the BHU.		-Refer only the most complex cases that can be treated on an outpatient basis; -Avoid referring patients who, despite being special, can be treated at the BHU, in order to make it easier for them to get around; and - In cases where sedation or general anesthesia is required, patients up to the age of 18 will be referred by the CEO to the Menino Jesus Hospital, while patients over this age will be referred to the Rocha Faria Hospital.

Source: prepared by the author as a summary of the protocols.

In the case of TMD, the oral environment must be adjusted beforehand and stomatology may refer you immediately.

With regard to knowledge of the existence of clinical protocols, six interviewees from primary care (85.7%) answered yes and only one DS (14.3%) reported not having any. Of those interviewed, five DCs (71.4%) said that these clinical protocols are used in their units, one DC (14.3%) said that they are not used and another DC (14.3%) reported not knowing.

When asked whether the oral health clinical protocol was important for referring patients from primary care to the DSC, the interviewees said the following:

"because we have guidance on how the service is organized" (PSIS3).

"because it sets standards for referrals" (PSIS2).

These statements demonstrate the importance of the protocols, which for the professionals have the function of organizing and standardizing referrals between the PHC and the DSC. This is corroborated by the Ministry of Health, when it states that the clinical protocols for BS, detailed in Chapter Five of Notebook 17 of the PHC Notebooks, contain recommendations for CRRs, in order to organize the flows between PHC and specialized care (BRASIL, 2004; BRASIL, 2006a).

With regard to the supply of appointments for specialties at the CEO, if they follow any criteria to organize the supply of vacancies, three (42.8%) of the CEO interviewees said they didn't know, one (14.4%) said they didn't and three (42.8%) said they did.

With regard to prioritization between different cases, one (14.3%) CEO professional said they didn't know, one (14.3%) said they didn't and the rest (71.4%) said they did.

Regarding the criteria for organizing vacancies and prioritizing different cases, the dentists interviewed said that there are pre-established priorities and criteria, as the following statements show:

"There are priorities from zero to three: zero is the need for immediate care; one is urgency or care as soon as possible; two is non-urgent priority; and three is elective care" (PSIS2).

"elements referred for endodontic treatment, for example, must follow pre-established criteria and must be restorable with the material offered at the AB" (PCEO7).

"Initially, vacancies are offered through SISREG on a weekly basis and the criteria are according to the protocols... the risk is taken by the regulator" (PCEO1).

"in the case of systematically compromised patients there is priority" (PCEO3).

The criteria established for referring patients from primary care to the DSC are those pre-defined in Notebook 17 of the primary care notebooks, which are the clinical protocols for referral.

Serra and Rodrigues (2010) state that among the elements that hinder patient access and the proper functioning of RCR systems is the low use of clinical protocols for referrals.

Rodrigues and Santos (2011) report that computer, telephone and radio communication systems must be agile, efficient, accessible to users, able to establish service priorities and controlled by management or regulatory centers.

The Smiling Brazil Program created a strategy to provide continuity and resolvability to the problems encountered in primary care. Thus, the CEOs are reference units with medium-complexity services, based on the guarantee of criteria identified for public access, based on the analysis of risk and user needs with the implementation of the RCR. This is how comprehensiveness is guaranteed in terms of user access and continuity of care (SILVA, 2009).

With regard to whether the referral form is filled in by hand or digitally, the permanent primary care DCs do it by hand, on the referral form, while those hired by the OSS (Health Organizations) do it digitally and print out the form to give to the patient.

Regarding the fact that filling in the referral form digitally brings benefits, all the primary care professionals were unanimous in saying that it did (100%):

"if it were digital it would be quicker to fill in the form and process" (PAB2).

"Yes, because it would speed up the work and registration process; the understanding of what is registered, even" (PAB5).

"Yes, because the documents wouldn't be lost, they would be archived, in other words, there would be a record" (PAB6).

From the analysis of these statements, it can be seen that digitization would bring benefits such as speeding up the work process, as well as corroborating the recording of documents, which is important for management.

Pimentel *et al* (2010) report that the faster and more reliable this referral is, the greater the chances of the patient following the correct referral flow.

In addition, the information and communication systems are precarious, which is why the most commonly used means of RCR is through paper forms. These deficiencies help us to understand the reduced resolubility of the services, which has implications for the health of the population (SERRA E RODRIGUES, 2010).

With regard to whether the referral form used was ideal and covered the necessary information, five (71.4%) DSC professionals considered that it was and agreed that there was no need to reformulate it. Only two (28.6%) professionals thought it was not and that it should be reformulated.

Regarding the suggested reformulations and the information that could be added:

"I think they could add other information, such as a priority field. Also, there's very little space to fill in" (PCEO2).

"I think there should be a field for the user's general status" (PAB4).

"the professional should write down the procedure carried out, which we often don't receive in the guide, and the patient's general health" (PSIS3).

"For me, there is a lack of ICD options to fit the patient and include the level of emergency or urgency of the case" (PAB5).

"I think it could include more information about the dental CID, as it is incomplete" (PAB7).

It can be seen from the comments that some professionals recommended reformulating the referral forms. They suggested adding a field to describe the patient's general condition, in order to differentiate between patients with different health conditions, which could in some way represent priority for care. In addition, they suggested expanding the options in the ICD (ANNEX), since they don't cover all the conditions needed to refer a patient from the PC to the DSC. It's worth noting that the ICD (International Classification of Diseases) is used to establish codes relating to the classification of diseases and health problems, identified throughout the world in a universal categorization.

According to the Ministry of Health, a distinction must be made between the conditions of risk and vulnerability, which prioritize the different cases of patients (BRASIL, 2011).

According to Serra (2003), comprehensiveness is related to the instruments of reference and counter-reference (RCR) and its guiding principle is continuity of care, which guarantees universal and equal access for users to primary care and other levels, according to the needs of each individual.

With regard to the operationalization of scheduling, the regulation of access in basic health is carried out by SISREG, which should guarantee or ensure access for patients from primary care to the secondary level:

"SB regulation is through SISREG, the computerized regulation system" (SB coordination).

When primary care professionals were asked whether the guarantee of access to the secondary level for continuity of care (integrality) is being covered by primary care, two DCs (28.5%) said no, while five (71.5%) said yes. On the same question, only one DC from the CEO (14.2%) answered yes, four (57.2%) answered no and two (28.6%) said they didn't know.

In this regard, the survey found deficiencies in the regulation process, such as insufficient numbers of professionals to meet demand, causing delays in scheduling and the unavailability of some specialties, as shown in the following statements:

"The number of specialties is not enough, for example, there are no prosthetics, orthodontics and others" (PAB5).

"I think it's taking longer and longer and the CEOs are becoming more and more bureaucratic" (PAB7).

"Comprehensiveness means having access to all your demands, in the sense of the patient's needs, but in the case of prostheses, it's still incipient or nil" (PCEO3).

"There is a demand and need for prostheses, which is not covered by the CEO... there is a lack of professionals to meet the ever-increasing demand of people who use AB" (PCEO6).

"Philosophically yes, but there is a lack of resources for integrality to be fully exercised in the SUS" (PCEO4).

"it is difficult for users to get to the CEO" (PCEO1).

"The main problems that hinder the regulation of referrals for consultations and exams are the lack of a specific professional for the regulation of referrals, the insufficient supply of specialized services, poor distribution of **CEOs** by programmatic area, absenteeism from consultations, lack of replacement of specialized professionals and lack of qualification and continuing education for these professionals.... there is greater transparency in the supply of vacancies and better organization of the system, but many points need to be reviewed and worked on to ensure that users have continuity of care for their needs... A crucial point is the expansion and qualification of secondary care" (SB coordination).

According to Mello *et al* (2014), with the implementation of DSCs, the structuring of medium complexity dentistry provided more complex procedures and allowed continuity of care for users without interrupting the oral health care line. Thus, the structuring of a reference center was considered a milestone in the development of an oral health care network.

However, the survey found some problems that hinder the regulation of referrals for specialized consultations and exams, and consequently represent a knot in the system, hindering the flow of patients from the PC to the DSC and ensuring continuity of care. Thus, the problems most frequently pointed out were the short supply of vacancies, which is insufficient to meet demand, caused by a lack of professionals in sufficient numbers, and the lack of some specialties that are also important for meeting the needs of the population.

In addition to basic care, the DSCs offer endodontics; specialized periodontics; minor oral surgery; stomatology; care for patients with special needs; preventive and interceptive orthodontics; and total and partial resin prostheses (RIO DE JANEIRO, 2013). However, it can be seen that orthodontic and prosthetic services are not available at the DSC studied, thus failing to meet the needs of users in this territory. This fact must be taken into account by the manager in order to guarantee the principle of comprehensiveness.

Ordinance No. 2.488 of 2011, issued by the Ministry of Health, states that comprehensive care is conditioned by supply, which, if insufficient, results in a waiting list, something considered to be the main problem for integration, contradicting what is recommended by the PNAB when it says that access to other levels of care must be under the right conditions, at the right time and with equity.

According to Mello *et al* (2014), most dental care in the SUS has been restricted almost solely to primary care and with a large pent-up demand, reflecting the country's social inequalities in the use of dental services. In 2000, according to the MS, secondary care had a low percentage, only 3.3%, within the scope of dental procedures. The lack of specialized services compromises the efficiency of the RCR in Oral Health. These facts culminated in the federal government's concern to encourage the creation of CEOs within the PNSB.

Another aspect analyzed that hinders regulation concerns the difficulty of access:

"it is difficult for users to get to the CEO" (PCEO1).

"The main problems that hinder the regulation of referrals for consultations and exams are... poor distribution of CEOs by programmatic area," (SB coordination).

The statements show that it is difficult for users to get to the DSC, which is often far away from the patient's place of residence, causing them to spend more on tickets, which makes it impossible for them to access the secondary level, jeopardizing continuity of care. This fact reveals the lack of planning for the distribution of DSCs by programmatic area, which shows that this sizing is done inadequately and randomly, without being based on the needs of users.

Serra and Rodrigues (2010) stated, based on the results of their research, that the provision of services continues to be geared towards meeting spontaneous demand and not the real needs of the population, based on epidemiological criteria.

In addition, the concept of offering services means that these services are accessible to the community and meet their health needs. The authors report that the concept of comprehensiveness is provided for by the 1988 Constitution as a guideline and as a principle by the LOS, as it refers to users' right of access to the actions of the different levels of complexity, with spatially defined and organized flows ensuring continuity of care in units located as close as possible to citizens. Thus, the units at each level of care must be sized in such a way as to guarantee the provision of services of sufficient quantity and quality. The main problems in referral, according to the same authors, are the limited supply of consultations and exams and the poor organization of regulation, as well as the difficulty of access due to financial problems, such as the cost of tickets.

However, the mere existence or availability of a service does not guarantee accessibility. For this reason, according to the authors, it is necessary to subdivide this concept into geographical accessibility - distance, travel time and means of transport; financial accessibility - payments or contributions for using services should not represent obstacles; cultural accessibility - there should be no conflict between the technical and administrative standards of the services and the habits, cultural standards and customs of the communities; and functional accessibility - the services should be provided in a timely and continuous manner, available at all times in order to meet real demand under a reference system that ensures easy access (BORGHI *et al*, 2013).

With regard to improving or speeding up the regulation of vacancies, the SB coordinator spoke about some initiatives:

"a new professional assisting in the regulation of SB, the creation of a whatsap group between professionals, specialists and managers, a request to the local coordination for the replacement of retired professionals and an increase in this specialized offer in the CEOs of area 3.1" (SB coordination).

Subcategory: training and continuing education

With regard to patients referred from primary care to the DSC arriving with properly filled out referral forms, only one DSC CD (14.3%) said no, while the others (85.7%) said yes.

Regarding the difficulty of filling it in and the most common errors, it was found that:

"There are bureaucratic doubts, such as which unit it comes from or goes to" (PCEO2).

"The professionals don't report what has already been done... often the dentist's name isn't legible. They also refer patients with teeth that are no longer suitable for endodontics" (PCEO6).

From these statements, it is clear that some professionals do not fill in the referral forms properly, without paying attention to the clinical protocols defined by the PHC Notebooks and this demonstrates the need to invest in training and capacity building for the team.

In relation to this report, Serra and Rodrigues (2010) found that the lack or deficiency of clinical protocols and referrals with little support from clinical protocols and guidelines reveals the need for continuing education programs.

In addition, the ineligibility of some of the data on the form reinforces the benefits of digitizing the process. This is reinforced by the study by the same authors, who found that information and communication systems are precarious, as there is a lack of networked telephones and computers, electronic medical records and systems for scheduling appointments and exams. As a result, paper forms are the most commonly used means of RCR. This deficiency is detrimental to comprehensiveness and continuity of care (SERRA E RODRIGUES, 2010).

As to whether the team had received any training on how to fill in the referral forms for the DSC based on the clinical protocols, six interviewees from primary care (85.7%) said they had not and only one DS (14.3%) said they had.

Regarding the need or importance of this staff training, the professionals said:

"This training is very important to promote the standardization of work in the team" (PAB1).

"by training the team, errors or doubts in filling in the application would be avoided and there would be uniformity in filling it in" (PAB5).

"It's important to standardize the way people are referred, the criteria for referral, like a standardization of the work processes of the dental team itself" (PAB6).

"It's important that the dentist, his assistants and technicians know how to do this regulation, because any mistake means that it has to be repeated and the patient is put on the waiting list once again" (PAB7).

"training on how to fill in the form is extremely important in order to standardize the format" (PAB3).

"This training is important because we would all be speaking the same language and would be better able to make these referrals correctly" (PAB4).

"the need for this training is to standardize the filling out of this form" (PSIS2).

"I think that perhaps this would bring a better understanding to the PC professional" (PSIS1).

"training would be important to avoid mistakes" (PSIS4).

"patients who are referred to the wrong specialty, the error is pointed out and referral to the correct specialty is requested" (PCEO1).

"the training allows us to fill out the form correctly, which will improve the flow of patients" (PCEO4).

"It is important to constantly update and evaluate the protocols of the specialties and to continuously disseminate them to the primary network, through constant training" (SB coordination).

It can be seen in these statements that the importance of training is noted by professionals from all the categories interviewed, including the OH coordination team. It stems from the fact that it trains all the professionals who make up the work team to properly fill out the referral forms, aiming for standardization and uniformity in order to correctly refer patients, allowing for an adequate flow and guaranteeing continuity of patient care.

When asked about the existence of a permanent education program (PEP) for primary care, five professionals (71.4%) said that it didn't exist and only two DCs (28.6%) said that it did. With regard to the same question for DSC professionals, six (85.7%) said it didn't exist and only one (14.3%) said it did. In this respect, the survey obtained the following statements:

"Yes, but this program only happens occasionally" (PAB5).

"There are a few sporadic meetings to discuss and solve problems of situational importance" (PAB7).

it only happens when there's a problem to solve" (PCEO2).

It can be seen that the interviewees report that the programs take place sporadically, without due regularity, only to solve specific problems, which does not contribute to the development of the actions.

Regarding the importance of this program, there was unanimity among all the interviewees (100%) from the PC and the CEO, who agreed that it was important, as shown in the statements below:

"it's important for constant updating" (PCEO6).

"it's important for updating network professionals" (PCEO7).

"I believe that constant updating is essential for professionals to perform adequately and safely" (PCEO4).

"The PNAC CEO has offered training in the specialties of TMD, stomatology and surgery, with in-house professionals as well as guests from outside the network, and we are involved in four research projects involving PNAC specialists in the areas of TMD, stomatology and endodontics" (PCEO1).

"episodic, sporadic courses, from time to time, would be interesting" (PCEO3).

"It would be interesting for the patients to understand better and for the professionals to understand better too, the referral criteria, in order to refer better and facilitate the work routine" (PCEO2).

"Another factor is the high level of absenteeism, which needs to be clarified and combated through permanent education of the population" (SB coordination).

Analyzing the statements, once again it can be seen that all the professionals, from both the PHC and the DSC, consider it important for the team to be trained on a regular basis, in order to improve the level of knowledge of the professionals, in a continuous process of updating and seeking knowledge, which also facilitates the daily practice of working together with the other professionals who make up the team and with the user, who in turn is an integral part of this learning process. In fact, the Health Coordination itself said that there is training for professionals in the use of the protocols established for referrals and sees the need to invest in courses in the areas of health surveillance, public health management and the use of information technology.

It is worth remembering that "permanent health education" is both a "teaching-learning practice" and a "health education policy":

As a 'teaching-learning practice', it means the production of knowledge in the daily life of health institutions, based on the reality experienced by the actors involved, with the problems faced in the day-to-day work and the experiences of these actors as the basis for questioning and change. Permanent health education' is based on the concept of 'problematizing teaching' (critically inserted in reality and without the educator's superiority over the student) and 'meaningful learning' (interested in the students' previous experiences and personal experiences, in other words, teaching and learning based on the production of knowledge that answers questions that belong to the universe of experiences of those who learn and that generate new questions about being and acting in the world (CECCIM & FERLA, 2009, s/p).

Thus, the PEP is a fundamental factor in the construction of the SUS, which seeks to articulate teaching, work and citizenship.

With regard to clinical management, the lack or deficiency of clinical protocols and referrals with little support from clinical protocols and guidelines reveals the need for ongoing education programs. With regard to human resources, it was observed that the lack of appropriate training for the function and the precariousness of continuing education contribute to the inadequate functioning of the RCR, which causes damage to the integrality and continuity of care, which are fundamental for the consolidation of the SUS (SERRA E RODRIGUES, 2010).

Subcategory: communication and information resources

- Communication between professionals

When asked about the existence of communication between professionals at the different levels of care, six (85.7%) of the interviewees from primary care reported that there was no such communication, just as there is no discussion of how to deal with the clinical case of patients who are referred to the CEO. Only one (14.3%) interviewee reported that there is communication between professionals.

As for the professionals at the CEO, three (42.8%) of the interviewees reported that there were none, just as there is no discussion of the conduct of the clinical case of patients who are referred to the CEO, while the other four (57.2%) said that there is.

On the communication channel between CEO and AB professionals:

"It's through the CAP, via the oral health accessory of AP 3.1" (PCEO1).

"the communication channel is via counter-reference" (PCEO6).

"communication is done through the referral and counter-referral guides" (PCEO6).

Regarding the importance of interaction between professionals at different levels of care:

"It would be of great importance, because the people who monitor these users are the CDS of primary care, so we could have a more detailed diagnosis and thus a more effective treatment" (PAB4).

"Integration between dentists is important to define the best course of action for each case" (PAB3).

"Communication is only with the CAP to answer questions about regulation... it would be very important to discuss clinical cases in order to better decide on treatment planning" (PAB7).

"Unfortunately, there is no such interaction. There should be, because it would be interesting to discuss clinical cases in order to find the best approach" (PAB5).

"discussing the case is important in order to establish a more resolute approach in certain cases" (PCEO7).

"there should be an opportunity to discuss conduct and reach unanimity" (PCEO2).

"more satisfactory and comprehensive care for patients and an exchange of knowledge between professionals" (PCEO4).

"the importance prevails in order to streamline and resolve the therapeutic conducts of patients, both in primary care and in the CEO, and thus we also have contact with tertiary care, since we refer these patients to this level of care" (PCEO1).

"It generates benefits for the end result, which is the patient, and learning among colleagues, who are the professionals" (PCEO3).

Regarding the importance of this interaction between professionals, the SB coordinator said the following:

"Certainly, this coordination is very important for the continuity of care... today, we have made the WhatsApp group available, coordinated by the advisors, as a tool to improve this coordination... we are raising the possibility of resuming the meetings" (SB coordination).

It can be seen from the interviewees from primary care, the DSC and the coordination of health care that there has not been adequate interaction between the professionals from the different levels of care, which they believe is important for discussing behavior, with a view to better planning and thus more effective treatment for the user. The professionals reported that the means of communication that has usually been used is through the referral and counter-referral guide, without there being a more effective interaction between the professionals.

With regard to human resources, it was observed that there is isolation among the professionals working in some units, according to Serra and Rodrigues (2010). In addition, the information and communication systems are precarious, as there is a lack of telephones, networked computers and electronic medical records. For this reason, the most commonly used means of RCR is through paper forms. From this we can understand the reduced resolubility of the program, which has implications for the health of the population.

- **Regular meeting**

Regarding the existence of a periodic meeting between the PC and the DSC professionals to discuss problems, difficulties and reformulate actions, all (100%) of the PC professionals reported that this did not exist. With regard to the CEO's DCs, only one (14.3%) professional said it existed and that it took place on a weekly basis. All the others (85.7%) said it didn't.

In fact, the following statement reveals that these meetings only take place to resolve specific cases, without any periodicity:

"meetings only take place when there is a specific problem to be resolved" (PAB6).

It can therefore be seen that there has not been adequate interaction between professionals from the different levels of care to discuss problems, difficulties and reformulate actions, with a view to better planning and thus a more effective and efficient service, with the user as the main beneficiary. Meetings take place only sporadically to resolve specific problems, with no pre-established frequency and no intention of reformulating the actions taken. In fact, the SB coordinator said:

"systematic meetings between subsystems must be re-established, which facilitate coordination between the health care network" (SB coordination).

With regard to interaction between professionals, Serra and Rodrigues (2010) referred to the isolation of professionals working in small units and without technical support, which contributes to the inadequate functioning of the RCR.

With regard to the reformulation of actions, Bulgarelli *et al* (2013) believe that it is important to evaluate oral health care models, guiding the planning and execution of actions, which is essential for building a more resolutive public dentistry, with greater efficiency and quality, realizing the principles of the SUS, especially in relation to integrality in health care networks.

- **Electronic Records**

The professionals who make up the ESB work with electronic medical records, while the statutory professionals do not have this tool. Regarding its importance for the coordination of primary care and the CEO:

"There is no articulation, because I don't see the CEO's information, nor does the CEO see my information" (PAB7).

"we don't use electronic medical records in primary care, but we do use them in conjunction with the CEO" (PAB4).

"If we had electronic medical records, it would be interesting to follow up and monitor requests, such as referrals for endodontic treatment of the patient's tooth" (PAB5).

"Electronic medical records would be important, because it would speed up the work process and there would be no loss of information about the patient" (PAB6).

"it's important because it optimizes the whole work process" (PAB3).

"It would be easier to integrate the specialties; you could follow the patient's history, where they come from and where they go" (PCEO2).

"The family clinics, the mixed units with ESB, yes, but the CEOs still don't have them... some don't even have a computer for the SB... the existence of a single electronic medical record, with access to the professionals of the primary and specialized care, would facilitate follow-up and better care for the user's integral health... the CEOs don't have a networked computer, nor do they have an electronic medical record.... I believe that it would speed up the user's journey through the network and reduce the risk of not understanding the procedures carried out, as they depend on the professional's handwriting... as for initiatives to improve coordination between primary and secondary care, the existing means of network communication between professionals should be maintained and improved" (SB coordination).

Analyzing the interviewees' statements, it can be seen that the professionals consider the use of electronic medical records to be relevant, since it allows them to record information about the patient, makes it possible to monitor them within the network, speeds up the work process, as well as enabling coordination between the PHC and the DSC. Another important point would be to make it easier for professionals to understand what is recorded, since the writing is digitalized and not manual. However, the ESB professionals who use the electronic medical record said that there is no such interaction, because the information recorded by the PC is not made available to the professionals at the DSC, and there is only an exchange of information between the professionals at the unit itself.

According to Ordinance No. 2,488 of 2011, issued by the Ministry of Health, which approved the PNAB, the transfer of information is fundamental to the regulation and continuity of care and, therefore, the importance of electronic medical records.

According to Giovanella *et al* (2009), long waiting lists are seen as the main problem in integrating the network. Managers recognize computerized units and electronic medical records as a major challenge to integrating the network and guaranteeing access to specialized care, as well as the availability and transfer of information, as these are essential for regulation and continuity of care. When they are not present, there is what is known as fragmentation of the system.

Serra and Rodrigues (2010) talked about the deficient information systems, such as medical records and electronic systems for scheduling appointments and specialized exams, which hinder the effective functioning of the RCR.

Category: counter-referral

In this category, the research analyzed and discussed the counter-referral flow from the Dental Specialty Center (CEO).

There was unanimity among all those interviewed (100%) about the existence of a standard counter-referral form. After the patient has been discharged from the specialty, the DC of the DSC sends the patient back to their UAB of origin, via counter-referral, in order to guarantee the continuity of the care that was started there. It is worth remembering that, according to Giovanella and Mendonça (2008), PHC must guarantee access to the various levels of care, with referral mechanisms for continuity of care and coordination of actions, which are interrelated and interdependent processes.

Regarding the fact that the counter-referral forms are always filled in, six (85.7%) AB interviewees answered yes and only one (14.3%) answered no.

"Every specialist is obliged to return the patient on discharge from the specialty, with the counter-referral, putting their name in a book and the patient signs it. This is done at the PNAC CEO" (PCEO1).

In the previous statement, it can be seen that the DSC registers the patient after discharge and makes a counter-referral to the PHC, which is important for achieving comprehensiveness, in the sense of continuity of care.

This fact is supported by Pimentel *et al* (2010), who say that ideally, after the end of treatment, the patient should be referred to the health unit of origin for the conclusion of treatment and maintenance, with the counter-referral form duly filled in, which should include the identification of the professional, the diagnosis and the treatment carried out.

In addition, among the important characteristics for the interconnection between primary and secondary care in the dental area is efficient and appropriate referral with counter-referral to primary care at the end of specialized treatment and easy return to secondary care whenever necessary. Failure to return patients from the DSC is an obstacle to comprehensiveness, as there is no continuity of care. The specialist professional must be committed to counter-referral and, above all, to informing patients of the importance of this return in concluding the case (BORGHI *et al*, 2013).

Of those interviewed, four professionals (57.1%) from the UBS considered that the DSC professionals did not fill in this form properly, two professionals (28.6%) considered that they did and only one professional (14.3%) reported not knowing. Another important point was that despite the counter-referral forms being filled in most of the time, the survey found that 57.1% of PHC professionals reported that they were not filled in properly.

When asked if they had any difficulty filling in the forms, four (57.2%) interviewees from the CEO said no, while three (42.8%) said yes. With regard to the existence of training on how to fill in the counter-referral forms, only one CEO DC (14.3%) answered yes, while all the others (85.7%) interviewed said they had not received any.

Regarding whether the counter-referral form is filled out by hand or digitally, all the professionals at the CEO (100%) were unanimous in saying that it is done by hand. When asked if filling in the form digitally would bring benefits, five (71.4%) CEO professionals said no, one (14.3%) said it was indifferent and one (14.3%) said yes.

When asked about the existence of special recommendations to be given to patients who are counter-referred to primary care, three (42.8%) interviewees from the CEO said no, while the other four (57.2%) said yes. When asked in which situations, the following statements follow:

"in some cases that require continued preservation" (PCEO3).

"I ask patients who have had a tooth treated endodontically to return to the AB and ask for the element to be restored straight away. Many clinicians do other teeth and leave this one until last, which often leads to fracture of the element" (PCEO6).

"**The** need to accompany the patient for clinical and radiographic assessments. There's nothing about it, but I write it down when I need to" (PCEO6).

"teeth with problems that trigger TMD or more urgent medical problems, such as those related to neurology and psychiatry" (PCEO2).

The importance of appropriate referrals from the DSC to the UAB can therefore be seen, where the specialist DS must be concerned with describing the conduct carried out and making any recommendations he deems important for the case, so that the patient can have their care continued appropriately by the PHC. In this context, Borghi *et al* (2013) emphasize that comprehensive care is the coordination of care by PHC, integrated into the network at other levels of care, ranging from access to resolving existing health needs on an ongoing basis.

As for the average turnaround time for patients referred from the DSC to the PC, the times varied from three to a maximum of eight months, according to the PC professionals. The specialty requiring the longest waiting time was endodontics, for five professionals (71.4%) of the seven primary care DCs interviewed.

It can be seen, then, that there is a delay in the return to the UAB of origin of patients referred to the CEO, and this is a consequence of the delay in scheduling the referred specialty.

Another important point is the follow-up of the referred patient, who often does not return to the unit of origin for follow-up and/or completion of treatment. Ideally, once the treatment is finished, the patient should be referred back to the health unit of origin for treatment completion and maintenance. (PIMENTEL *et al,* 2010).

When asked about the BHU's conduct after the return of the counter-referred patient, the PHC professionals were unanimous (100%) in answering that they schedule the patient immediately. This is a positive aspect, which helps ensure continuity of care for the patient.

It should be noted that according to Borghi *et al* (2013), counter-referral is deficient when the majority of patients do not return to the UAB of origin. According to the authors, the interconnection between primary and secondary care in the dental field should allow patients to be referred efficiently and appropriately, with counter-referral, to primary care at the end of the specialized treatment, as well as easily returning to secondary care whenever necessary.

Silva (2009) also considers that in order to truly achieve comprehensiveness, in the sense of guaranteeing continuity of care in order to solve the user's health needs, the RCR system must be the link between the user and the other levels of care, allowing them to go through the entire system according to their needs and always return to the point of origin, which is primary care.

With regard to counter-referrals, the SB Coordination took this position:

"PHC professionals are instructed to coordinate care with their patients, explaining the importance of them returning as soon as possible to the unit of origin, with the counter-referral guide, for continuity of care" (SB coordination).

Based on this statement, it can be seen that the coordination department says it has made an effort to ensure that primary care professionals advise their patients on the need to return to the unit with a counter-referral form as soon as they have completed their treatment by the specialist at the CEO, in order to continue the care they started there.

Category: potential and weaknesses for access

Through the analysis of this category, the potential and weaknesses for access to dental specialties were identified. In order to facilitate understanding, the main points made by all the participants in the survey were highlighted:

- **Potential:**

1)   SISREG is an organizer and guarantor of access to the CEO.

Patients are referred from the UBS to the CEO via the regulation system (SISREG). Thus, the CEO offers the vacancy in the specialty to the regulation center, which notifies the UBS:

"The primary care unit refers the patient to the CEO, through SISREG, which regulates the vacancies... the CEO makes the vacancies available weekly to the regulation center, which will notify the unit that referred the patient to a certain specialty" (PCEO1).

"The dentist refers the patient to a specialty, such as endodontics, surgery, stomatology, etc. Then I enter the request or need in SISREG... then the regulation center notifies us when a vacancy arises at the CEO for that specialty, giving the day and time of the appointment, and we call to tell the patient about the appointment at the CEO" (PSIS1).

Thus, in everyday practice, users are seen in primary care and, after all therapeutic possibilities have been exhausted, they are referred for specialized care at the CEO. This process is regulated through a computerized system which, according to the Ministry of Health, aims to guarantee access to exams, specialist consultations and hospitalizations at the most complex levels by referring patients (BRASIL, 2006b).

2) The regulatory system lists priorities.

The referral of patients from the PHC to the DSC follows the pre-defined criteria of Notebook 17 of the PHC notebooks and there is prioritization between different cases:

"in the case of systematically compromised patients there is priority" (PCEO3).

"There are priorities from zero to three: zero is the need for immediate care; one is urgency or care as soon as possible; two is non-urgent priority; and three is elective care" (PSIS2).

Referral to secondary care is based on an analysis of the user's risk and needs (SILVA, 2009).

Rodrigues and Santos (2011) report that the management or regulation centers must be able to control and organize, but also to establish service priorities.

3) The availability of specialized services in the public network (previously there were only services and actions related to primary care).

The PNAC CEO is a reference for all the AB units on Ilha do Governador and has the following specialties: Periodontics, Endodontics, TMD, Minor Oral Surgery, Stomatology and Care for Patients with Special Needs:

"As I've been working in primary care for a long time, I'm very happy to see the possibility of having a patient referred for a root canal, which used to be impossible... I could only extract the tooth" (PAB6).

"guarantees specialized care... allows the maintenance of elements that would otherwise be removed" (PAB3).

"It filled a gap in the network, because there was only AB" (PAB5).

Referrals to the DSC are made after all clinical resources in primary care have been exhausted. According to Campos *et al* (2010), PHC should be one of the main gateways to the health system, but much more is expected of it than just the function of guaranteeing access to the system, such as the ability to solve around 80% of problems while the remaining cases would be referred, thus making up an articulated network of services that expands the capacity to solve the patient's health problems in a comprehensive manner.

- Weaknesses:

1) Insufficient supply of specialized services (need to include other specialties, such as prosthetics and orthodontics).

On this issue, the research found some statements that show deficiencies in the regulation process, such as the unavailability of some specialties:

"The number of specialties is not enough, for example, there are no prosthetics, orthodontics and others" (PAB5).

"There is a need to include other specialties, such as orthodontics, since there are a huge number of children seen in primary care, many of them with malocclusions that could be prevented and even treated" (PAB6).

"Comprehensiveness means having access to all your demands, in the sense of the patient's needs, but in the case of prostheses, it's still incipient or nil" (PCEO3).

"there is a demand and need for prostheses, which is not covered by the CEO... there is a lack of professionals to meet the ever-increasing demand of people who use AB" (PCEO6).

In addition to basic care, the DSCs offer endodontics; specialized periodontics; minor oral surgery; stomatology; care for patients with special needs; preventive and interceptive orthodontics; and total and partial resin prostheses (RIO DE JANEIRO, 2013). However, it can be seen that orthodontic and prosthetic services are not available at the DSC studied, thus failing to meet the needs of users in this area. This fact must be taken into account by the manager in order to guarantee the principle of comprehensiveness.

2) Insufficient supply of specialized professionals.

The survey also found some problems that cause a knot in the system, hindering the flow of patients from the PC to the DSC and ensuring continuity of care. Thus, among the most pointed out problems were the short supply of vacancies, which is insufficient to meet demand, caused by a lack of sufficient professionals:

"The main problems that make it difficult to regulate referrals for consultations and exams are the lack of a specific professional to regulate referrals, the insufficient supply of specialized services, poor distribution of CEOs by program area, absenteeism from consultations, lack of replacement of specialized professionals..." (SB coordination).

Ordinance 2.488 of 2011, issued by the Ministry of Health, states that comprehensive care is conditioned by supply which, if insufficient, results in a waiting list, considered to be the main problem for integration, contradicting what is recommended by the PNAB when it says that access to other levels of care must be under the right conditions, at the right time and with equity.

3)   Delays in scheduling (large number of users waiting for appointments) CEO).

What has been observed in the interviewees' statements is that there is a delay in scheduling users of the health system, due to the disproportion between the supply of services and the demand for patients, causing queues:

"the patient waited so long that when he arrived at the CEO, the element was already out of protocol" (PAB4).

"Here, patients always prefer to have a private scan, because it's a cheap test that patients can afford, and it's quicker, because you don't have to wait for a SISREG slot" (PSIS1).

"this is justified by the length of time the patient has to wait in line" (PCEO7).

"There has been an expansion of the ESF, but on the other hand there is a lack of incentive and resources for the CEO... because there is a lot of pent-up demand" (PCEO1).

According to Giovanella *et al* (2009), SISREG should make it possible to book specialized exams and consultations immediately, with a sufficient supply.

4)   Absenteeism (due to scheduling delays).

The delay in scheduling appointments in secondary care sometimes leads to absenteeism. According to the Health Coordination, the waiting lists are monitored and this problem is being tackled:

"through the management of lists by the head of the DSC and the periodic analysis of data regarding appointments, absenteeism... the main problems that hinder the regulation of referrals for consultations and exams are the lack of a specific professional for the regulation of referrals, the insufficient supply of specialized services, the poor distribution of DSCs by programmatic area, absenteeism from consultations, the lack of replacement of specialized professionals and the lack of training and continuing education for these professionals..." (SB coordination).

According to Giovanella *et al* (2009), SISREG should monitor the user's journey, thus reducing the number of absentees.

5)   Distance (inaccessibility) and poor distribution of CEOs by program area.

Referral via SISREG to units outside the Ilha do Governador neighborhood sometimes leads to users giving up due to the distance and cost of travel:

"When you need an X-ray, I refer you through SISREG, which gives you a place at another CEO, off the island, and that's why most patients prefer to go to a private clinic, right here in the neighborhood, because it's cheaper and easier than leaving the island" (PSIS1).

This situation has already been studied by authors such as Serra and Rodrigues (2010), who found that the proper functioning of the RCR is compromised by a lack of planning, which in this case refers to the poor spatial distribution of the units.

6)   Lack of training, continuing and permanent education for professionals (professionals not adequately trained).

It is clear that some professionals do not fill in the referral forms properly, without paying attention to the clinical protocols defined by the PHC guidelines, and this demonstrates the need to invest in training the team. With regard to the difficulty in filling in the forms and the most common errors, the following statements were made:

"The professionals don't report what has already been done... often the dentist's name isn't legible. They also refer patients with teeth that are no longer suitable for endodontics" (PCEO6).

"It often seems that the dentists at the PHC don't know how to proceed with the patient and refer them to the CEO to save time... cases such as supra-gingival scraping, which are often sent unnecessarily to the CEO" (PCEO6).

"because these professionals must be prepared to carry out their activities and if we don't receive this training, the work becomes more complicated and sometimes we run into difficulties" (PSIS4).

Serra and Rodrigues (2010) found in a study that, in terms of human resources, there was a lack of appropriate training for the job and precarious continuing education.

7)   Lack of resources or investment in secondary care, which has not kept pace with the expansion of the ESF (which has increased repressed demand).

The study found that the expansion of the ESF has not been accompanied by secondary care, which lacks supplies, equipment, replacement and training of professionals, insufficient specialties, among other deficiencies. There is a shortage of human and material resources, which leads to discontinuity in health care:

"Philosophically yes, but there is a lack of resources for integrality to be fully exercised in the SUS" (PCEO4).

"There has been an expansion of the ESF, but on the other hand there is a lack of incentive and resources for the CEO... because there is a lot of pent-up demand... there has been an increase in pent-up demand for the ESF, which has not kept up with the lack of resources for the polyclinics... unfortunately the city has forgotten about the polyclinics" (PCEO1).

"With the expansion of primary care in the municipality, the increase in the population covered and the family clinics, our secondary care network has not received any specialized professionals, which would increase the supply of specialized vacancies... through a survey of SISREG reports and monitoring with the DSCs, we were able to justify to the local coordination the need to bring in some specialized professionals, such as periodontists,... to our DSCs. to our CEOs" (SB coordination).

According to Vilarinho, Mendes and Prado Júnior (2007), the expansion of the secondary and tertiary care network has not kept pace with the growth in the supply of primary care services in the dental sector.

For Aquilante and Aciole (2015), the integration of services is one of the most serious impediments to comprehensive health care, since comprehensive actions are restricted to the USF. Thus, when actions are needed at other levels of complexity, the system is vulnerable, as it does not respond satisfactorily to the user's needs.

8)   Bureaucracy.

The survey found that there are difficulties when it comes to filling in referral forms. There are professionals who do not fill in these forms properly, and this again demonstrates the need to invest in training and capacity building for the team.

"There are bureaucratic doubts, such as which unit it comes from or goes to" (PCEO2).

"The professionals don't report what has already been done... often the dentist's name isn't legible. They also refer patients with teeth that are no longer suitable for endodontics" (PCEO6).

"PHC has improved a lot in recent years, but bureaucracy is still a barrier... there is an exacerbated delay that sometimes makes treatment unfeasible... the patient often returns to the referral unit reporting that he has not been called and when he consults SISREG, the situation is pending" (PSIS1).

For Aquilante and Aciole (2015), the established protocols are still being appropriated by professionals. When analyzing the RCR process, the authors found that it is limited to bureaucratic issues.

9)   Lack of communication and information.

Analyzing what was said by the interviewees, it can be seen that the professionals consider it important to invest in communication and information resources, such as the use of electronic medical records, since this makes it possible to record information about the patient, monitor them within the network, speed up the work process, as well as making it possible to link the PHC and the DSC. Another important point would be to make it easier for professionals to understand what is recorded, since the writing is digitalized and not manual. However, the ESB professionals, who use the electronic medical record, reported that there is no such interaction, as the information recorded by the PC is not made available to the CEO professionals, and there is only an integration between the professionals of the unit itself:

"If we had electronic medical records, it would be interesting to follow up and monitor requests, such as referrals for endodontic treatment of the patient's tooth" (PAB5).

"It would be easier to integrate the specialties; you could follow the patient's history, where they come from and where they go" (PCEO2).

"The family clinics, the mixed units with ESB, yes, but the CEOs still don't have them... some don't even have a computer for the SB... the existence of a single electronic medical record, with access to primary care and specialized professionals, would facilitate follow-up and better care for the user's comprehensive health... the CEOs don't have a networked computer, nor do they have an electronic medical record.... I believe it would speed up the user's journey through the network and reduce the risk of not understanding the procedures carried out, as they depend on the professional's handwriting... as for initiatives to improve coordination between primary and secondary care, the existing means of network communication between professionals should be maintained and improved" (SB coordination).

According to Serra and Rodrigues (2010), the information and communication systems are precarious, as there is a lack of telephones, networked computers and electronic medical records. For this reason, paper forms are the most commonly used means of RCR. From this we can understand the reduced resolubility of the Program and the inadequate functioning of the RCR.

10)   Rigid criteria or inflexibility of referral protocols - rigid, old and limited protocols.

The protocols recommended and adopted in practice by the units are those proposed by the Ministry of Health in accordance with Notebook 17 of the PHC Notebooks. The study identified numerous restrictions contained in the specialty protocols, which must be followed by UBS dentists in order to refer their patients to the CEO's specialties. If these protocols are not applied, the patient will be excluded from the possibility of treatment in secondary care, which often means more radical and even mutilating treatment:

"The elements referred for endodontic treatment, for example, must follow pre-established criteria and must be restorable with the material offered at AB" (PCEO7).

"Initially, vacancies are offered through SISREG on a weekly basis and the criteria are according to the protocols..." (PCEO1).

"Patients return to primary care without the services being carried out as they should be, for example, they come up against the rigidity of the protocol imposed by the network, as in the case of the difficulty of root canal treatment... I recommend making the referral protocol more flexible" (PAB5).

"the protocols for referrals are very rigid, limited and inflexible, excluding some clinical cases" (PAB6).

"too many clinical prerequisites for referral, such as the tooth must be intact to have a root canal" (PAB7).

"constantly updating and evaluating the protocols of the specialties and disseminating them to the primary care network through constant training" (SB coordination).

These statements show the importance of the protocols, which the professionals believe have the function of organizing and standardizing referrals between the PHC and the DSC. This is corroborated by the Ministry of Health, which states that the clinical protocols for BS, detailed in Chapter Five of Notebook 17 of the PHC Notebooks, contain recommendations for CRRs, in order to organize the flows between PHC and specialized care (BRASIL, 2004; BRASIL, 2006a).

Aquilante and Aciole (2015) reported that when actions at other levels of complexity are required, the system is vulnerable because it does not respond satisfactorily to the user's needs. In addition, there are established protocols that are still being appropriated by professionals, which shows that the RCR process is limited to bureaucratic issues. This, according to the authors, often ends up leaving users more vulnerable to future mutilating treatments.

Serra and Rodrigues (2010) note the importance of team training and continuing education programs, as it is essential to adapt to the user's reality or needs.

This leads us to reflect on the need to periodically re-evaluate the clinical protocols used in order to bring them up to date with the real needs of users in a given territory. They must not be rigid or rigid in a way that does not allow them to be adapted to the local reality. Hence the importance of making protocols more flexible.

When patients come up against the limitations set by the protocol, they are unable to have their problem solved by secondary care and often give up on treatment. What's more, most of the time these patients don't even return to primary care to continue their treatment.

Pimentel *et al* (2010) observed that patients who are referred often do not return to the unit of origin for maintenance or completion of treatment, when secondary care does not carry out the action or service it was supposed to, resulting in discontinuity of care.

Category: professionals' perceptions

This category allowed us to analyze the perception of the professionals involved in the process of consolidating integrality. The following subcategories were extracted: lack of professional knowledge, primary care as a gateway, expansion of coverage by the ESF and the need to invest in secondary care to guarantee comprehensiveness.

Subcategory: lack of professional knowledge

"I don't know what RAS is and I don't know the importance of integrating PC with RAS..." (PAB2).

"I understand that the ESF works by area, but I don't understand it very well... I understand very little about it, I just know that there's basic care, the CEO and high-complexity hospital care" (PCEO2).

An analysis of the speeches showed that there are professionals who are not fully aware of the structure of the health system, and in some cases are unaware of basic concepts about the different levels of care, the ESF, the RAS, comprehensiveness, and so on. This shows that there are professionals who are not trained and, in turn, the coordination has not been investing enough in training and continuing and permanent education for the professionals who make up the health network, in order to contribute to the process of consolidating integrality.

With regard to human resources, Serra and Rodrigues (2010) observed that the lack of appropriate training for the job and the precariousness of continuing education contribute to the inadequate functioning of the system and harm to comprehensiveness.

Subcategory: AB as a gateway

"PHC is fundamental because it is the gateway to other services and will continue the patient's line of care... PHC has to offer the patient all the procedures or services offered in the PHC booklet" (PAB5).

"The RAS would be the entire network of public health services offered to the population... primary care is fundamental, because it is the gateway to refer the patient to the other services" (PAB6).

"Primary care is the starting point for organization, so an organized primary care will be responsible for organizing the hierarchical process... The CEO is the divider between primary and tertiary care and will be responsible for triaging patients to the hospital network... comprehensiveness is care that begins in primary care and continues throughout the HCN" (PCEO1).

"Primary care is the basis of the network, the point of reference that articulates with the other levels of care... the CEO expands the resolutiveness of the SUS" (PSIS2).

"Primary care is very important... we are the first contact with the patient, we are the ones who welcome and diagnose... the implementation of the CEOs is equally important, since this is an extension of our service... Primary care has improved a lot in recent years, but bureaucracy is still a barrier... there is an exacerbated delay that sometimes makes treatment unfeasible... integrality is not being contemplated due to bureaucracy and delay" (PSIS1).

Professionals generally consider primary care to be the gateway to the system, and the fundamental axis for coordinating care. PHC is responsible for solving most of the patient's health problems, going as far as the clinic and when it is no longer able to solve them, it must refer the patient to the secondary level, which in SB is represented by the CEO, where medium-complexity dental services are provided.

According to the Ministry of Health, primary care is responsible for providing oral health care until all therapeutic possibilities have been exhausted at primary level. Then, when the possibility of treatment at this level of care is exceeded and more complex dental procedures are required, the patient is referred to the CEO (Dental Specialties Center) (BRASIL, 2004b).

Subcategory: expanding ESF coverage

"I see the ESF positively, because it focuses on primary care, prevention and health promotion" (PAB1).

"I think the concept of the ESF is good, but in practice I still see obstacles... the CEOs will carry out treatments that aren't available in primary care" (PAB2).

"the ESF is a proposal to reformulate and reorganize the system, through primary care as the main access to health, with a focus on prevention and promotion..." (PAB3).

"The ESF was the reorganization of primary care in order to increase resolution... comprehensiveness would be an integral and not partial condition for understanding the human being, in other words, the health system must be prepared to listen to the user, understand them in their social context and, from there, understand their demands and needs" (PAB4).

The speeches showed that the ESF has expanded population coverage and access to primary care, but that secondary care still does not receive enough resources to meet this increased demand, which causes obstacles in the flow of continuity of care, which should be continuous from primary care.

According to Oliveira and Pereira (2013), the organization of primary care, through the ESF, prioritizes actions to promote, protect and recover comprehensive health in a continuous manner, including practices and services that go beyond medical care and are based on the needs of the population, which are understood through the establishment of bonds between users and professionals. The ESF is centered on the family, perceived from its social and physical environment, as well as the living and health conditions of the population, allowing them a broader understanding of the health-disease process.

Subcategory: need to invest in secondary care to ensure comprehensiveness

"Comprehensiveness is for the person to start their care at the PHC and follow it up with other services in the network, if necessary, in case the PHC can't solve the problem. I think that comprehensiveness is partially guaranteed, because we don't have the number of specialists and services that would be necessary to meet the needs, for example, there are no prostheses or orthodontics in the network... patients return to primary care without the services being carried out as they should" (PAB5).

"Comprehensiveness is the person starting care in primary care and continuing care in the other services of the network. I don't think this right is guaranteed by either the PC or the DSC because patients return to the PC without the services being carried out as they should be... I think that unfortunately there is no guarantee of access to secondary care" (PAB6).

"The importance of integrating primary care with the other levels is the continuity of the service. It's important to know that the professional can count on specialists for care... the right to comprehensive care is guaranteed, because if necessary, the PHC can refer the patient to the DSCs and then return for review appointments at the PHC, but I think that care is taking longer and longer and is becoming more bureaucratic" (PAB7).

"Comprehensiveness means having access to all their demands, in the sense of the patient's needs... but in the case of prostheses it is still incipient or nil" (PCEO3).

"The CEO is fundamental in the process of implementing SB and quality of life, so that patients are fully satisfied with their health... the principle of comprehensiveness is guaranteed philosophically, but resources are lacking for comprehensiveness to be fully exercised in the SUS" (PCEO4).

"The CEO is essential for meeting more specific demands... not all rights are guaranteed by the CEO... there is a demand and need for prostheses that is not covered by the CEO" (PCEO6).

"To achieve comprehensiveness, it would be necessary to provide more specialists such as prosthetics and orthodontics" (PSIS2).

"The DSCs still leave something to be desired in terms of comprehensive patient care... it could be better because there are few vacancies and the demand is high." (PSIS4).

"There is greater transparency in the supply of places and better organization of the system, but many points need to be reviewed and worked on to ensure that users have continuity of care for their needs. A crucial point is the expansion and qualification of secondary care" (SB coordination).

The professionals interviewed agreed on the need to invest in secondary care so that it can be expanded, in the same way as primary care, in order to meet the needs of the population in a given territory. The statements show that there is a shortage of professionals and a lack of some specialties that are necessary for continuity of care, such as orthodontics and prosthetics.

For Aquilante and Aciole (2015), the integrality of the health system refers to the articulation of the different levels of care, so that users can move through the system and have their health needs met. On the other hand, the integration of services is one of the most serious impediments to comprehensive health care, since comprehensive actions are restricted to the USF. When actions at other levels of complexity are required, the system is vulnerable, as it does not respond satisfactorily to the user's needs.

These shortcomings have caused waiting lines, delays in seeing patients referred to the DSC, absenteeism and even patients returning to primary care without having their problem solved by secondary care. Therefore, according to the SB coordinator's own report, despite the progress made by the SUS in terms of expanding primary care and the provision of specialized services by the CEO, it is still necessary to invest in actions to really guarantee integrality, in the sense of continuity of care in SB, where the patient goes through the entire health system without hindrance, guaranteeing the user the right guaranteed by law to comprehensive health care.

According to Kuschnir and Chorny (2010), the organization of the integrated health system into care networks must guarantee continuity of care, as these systems are responsible for guaranteeing the right to health and regionalized networks as an instrument for expanding access and reducing inequalities. After all, this would provide health services for comprehensive care for the entire population of a region or territory, given that primary care would be the "gateway" to the system, with general practitioners and would be linked to the secondary level with the offer of specialized services.

Serra and Rodrigues (2010) report on the concept of comprehensiveness, provided for as a guideline by the Federal Constitution and as a principle by the LOS, which refers to the right of users to access the actions of the different levels of complexity, with defined and spatially organized flows in order to ensure continuity of care in units located close to the citizens. The integration of health networks is guaranteed by the effective RCR system, which establishes the mutual referral of patients between the different levels of complexity, since the Ministry of Health itself defines this system as one of the key elements in the reorganization of working practices.

7   Final considerations

This study analyzed three health units, two of which were primary care units and one secondary care unit, all located in the Ilha do Governador district, in the municipality of Rio de Janeiro, in an attempt to gain a better understanding of how integration between oral health services takes place in daily practice in this territory.

The Guidelines of the National Oral Health Policy of January 2004, implemented by the Smiling Brazil Program of March 17, 2004 (MS), led to increased access to oral health promotion, prevention and recovery actions, through the implementation of the ESB, which restructured the oral health model, now centered on the family through the ESF, with the proposal of improving the epidemiological indices of the Brazilian population, related to oral health conditions.

In addition, the program set up the CEOs, injecting resources to provide specialized dental services to complement the actions initiated by primary care, in order to make comprehensive oral health services possible.

The restructuring of dentistry in the municipality of Rio de Janeiro required investments to reorganize and expand primary care, which must have a high capacity to solve the population's health problems. At the same time, however, there was a need to invest in secondary care, since the expansion of primary care led to an increase in SUS users' need for specialized services.

In theory, these initiatives to widen access and increase the supply of basic services would bring great visibility to dentistry and, above all, benefits to the population. However, in practice, it has brought other problems related to oral health, which has ultimately shown that it would be necessary to invest more effectively in secondary care, in order to promote the expansion of the supply of specialized exams and services.

The CEOs were supposed to guarantee the specialized demands, based on the needs requested by the UBS. To this end, a central vacancy regulation system was set up through a computerized regulation system (SISREG), to organize or coordinate the referral and counter-referral system, through the Municipal Health Department together with the Oral Health Coordination.

Despite the municipality's efforts to regulate vacancies in a coordinated way, in order to meet the needs initiated by primary care, in order to provide comprehensive health care to the population of its territory, guaranteeing continuity of care, some difficulties have arisen in the municipality of Rio de Janeiro, as well as in the neighborhood studied.

With regard to the provision of BS services, the survey found that when the possibility of treatment in primary care is exceeded and more complex dental procedures are required, the patient is referred to the CEO, which on Ilha do Governador is located in the PNAC (Newton Alves Cardoso Polyclinic) and provides care in the following specialties: Periodontics, Minor Oral Surgery, Endodontics, Patients with Special Needs, Stomatology and TMD (Temporomandibular Disorder).

This shows that there is no provision of orthodontic or prosthodontic services, which in turn were mentioned in the survey as necessary services to meet the demand of users of oral health services in the territory studied. This shows that the supply of services is not planned from the point of view of meeting the needs of the population, as it should be, but according to the specialties available in the unit.

Endodontics was the specialty with the highest number of referrals, i.e. the highest demand. This should be taken into account by the manager when planning the supply of services, avoiding the occurrence of waiting lines caused by the disproportion between supply and demand. This runs counter to the SISREG proposal, which would make it possible to book specialized exams and consultations immediately, thanks to a sufficient supply.

When periapical radiography is needed to complement the diagnosis, a referral must be made via SISREG, and it is carried out in units outside the Ilha do Governador neighborhood. This leads to users giving up due to the waiting time, the distance and the cost of travel, thus leading them to carry out these examinations at clinics or private practices in their own neighborhood. In the case of panoramic X-rays, the referral unit is the Nossa Senhora do Loreto Municipal Hospital, which is located in the neighborhood itself. However, for this test to be carried out, the patient must also be referred via the Vacancy Regulation System, which, in most cases, leads the user to also opt for the private network due to the distance and delay in scheduling. Once again, the functioning of the RCR is compromised, demonstrating a lack of planning, which in this case refers to a random spatial distribution of the units.

The study found that vacancies are made available on a weekly basis by the CEO, but the number of vacancies is offered according to the availability of existing professionals and not according to patients' needs. The expansion of the ESF has led to an increase in the registered population, but has not increased the number of professionals, which has led to pent-up demand and a waiting list. This has compromised the integrality of the health system, where users can move freely and have their needs met through a continuous flow between primary care and the CEO.

With regard to the criteria adopted by dental surgeons for referring users registered at the Zumbi and Bancàrios units to the secondary unit, as well as the scheduling of specialized oral health appointments, the survey found that there is no informality when it comes to referring patients. There are defined formal structures in place, using prepared forms. It should be emphasized that it is essential to use referrals based on the protocols and clinical guidelines recommended by the

Ministry of Health, in accordance with Caderno 17 of the Cadernos da AB. Among the elements that hinder patient access and the proper functioning of RCR systems is the low use of clinical protocols for referrals.

The survey showed that some professionals do not fill out the referral forms properly, without paying attention to the clinical protocols, and this demonstrates the need to invest in training, staff qualification and continuing education programs. However, the interviewees report that the programs take place without due regularity, only to solve specific problems, which does not contribute to the development of actions, which causes damage to the integrality and continuity of care, which are fundamental for the consolidation of the SUS.

With regard to the operationalization of scheduling, the regulation of access in BS is carried out by SISREG, which should guarantee or ensure access for patients from primary care to the secondary level. The study found deficiencies in the regulation process, such as insufficient numbers of professionals to meet demand, causing delays in scheduling and the unavailability of some specialties. This goes against the initial proposal, which states that with the implementation of the CEOs, the structuring of medium complexity dentistry would provide more complex procedures and allow continuity of care for the user without interrupting the oral health care line.

The interviewees' statements show that there has not been adequate interaction between professionals at the different levels of care, and that they consider it important to discuss procedures, with a view to better planning and thus more **effective** treatment for the user. The professionals said that the means of communication that has usually been used is through the referral and counter-referral guide, without there being a more effective interaction between the professionals. Thus, the information and communication systems are precarious, as there is a lack of telephones, networked computers and electronic medical records. For this reason, paper forms are the most commonly used means of RCR. From this we can understand the reduced resolubility of the program, which has implications for the health of the population.

With regard to the counter-referral flow from the DSC, it was found that there is a standard counter-referral form. Thus, after the patient has been discharged from the specialty, the CD at the CEO sends the patient back to their UAB of origin, via counter-referral, in order to guarantee the continuity of the care that was started there. Ideally, once the treatment is finished, the patient should be sent back to the unit of origin to complete the treatment and maintenance, with the counter-referral form duly filled in, which should include the identification of the professional, the diagnosis and the treatment carried out.

The non-return of patients from the DSC is an obstacle to comprehensiveness, as there is no continuity of care. Therefore, the specialist professional must make an effort to make counter-referrals and, above all, to inform patients of the importance of returning for the conclusion of the case, as well as maintenance.

Another important point was that although the counter-referral forms are filled in most of the time, the survey found that in many cases they are not carried out satisfactorily, which could be solved by training the staff.

As for the average turnaround time for patients referred to the CEO for primary care, the times ranged from three to a maximum of eight months. The specialty that requires the longest waiting time was endodontics. This delay in returning to the UAB of origin is a consequence of the delay in scheduling for the referred specialty.

Regarding the BHU's behavior after the return of the counter-referred patient, the survey found that the patient is immediately scheduled. This is a positive aspect, which corroborates the guarantee of continuity of care for the patient. It's worth pointing out that, in order to truly achieve comprehensiveness, in the sense of guaranteeing continuity of care, the RCR system must be the link between the user and the other levels of care, allowing them to go through the whole system according to their needs and always return to the point of origin, which is primary care.

As for the strengths and weaknesses of access to dental specialties, the main points were highlighted, listed below:

Potential:

- SISREG is an organizer and guarantor of access to the CEO;

- The regulatory system lists priorities; and

- The availability of specialized services in the public network (previously there were only services and actions related to primary care)

Weaknesses:

- Insufficient supply of specialized services (need to include other specialties, such as prosthetics and orthodontics);

- Insufficient supply of specialized professionals;

- Delay in scheduling (large number of users waiting to be seen by the CEO);

- Absenteeism (due to scheduling delays);

- Distance from the CEO (inaccessibility) and poor distribution of CEOs by program area;

- Lack of training, continuing and permanent education for professionals (professionals not adequately trained);

- Lack of resources or investment in secondary care, which has not kept pace with the expansion of the ESF (which has increased repressed demand);

- Bureaucracy;

- Lack of communication and information; and

- Rigid criteria or inflexibility of referral protocols - rigid, old and limited protocols.

The research found, in general, that despite the positive aspects achieved through the implementation of medium-complexity dental services and the regulation of access through SISREG, there are still many fragile points that need to be tackled in order to guarantee continuity of care.

The survey of the perception of the professionals involved in the process of consolidating integrality revealed that there are professionals who do not have full knowledge of the structure of the health system, who are unaware of the basic concepts of the different levels of care, the ESF, the RAS, integrality, and so on. These professionals are not trained and, in turn, the management, despite all its efforts, recognizes that it has been insufficient in terms of training and continuing and permanent education, in order to contribute to the process of consolidating integrality.

The reports showed that the ESF has expanded the coverage of the registered population and their access to primary care. However, it has been noted that secondary care has not received sufficient resources to meet this increased demand, which has hampered the flow of care.

continuity of care that should be continuous from primary care. Thus, the integration of services is one of the most serious impediments to comprehensiveness, since comprehensive actions are restricted to the USF. When actions at other levels of complexity are required, the system is vulnerable, as it does not respond satisfactorily to the user's needs.

However, it is essential to point out that the progress that has already been made, despite some shortcomings, has allowed the district of Ilha do Governador and the municipality of Rio de Janeiro to restructure and reorganize health services. However, it has not yet been achieved that supply and demand are balanced and that users can have their right to continuity of care guaranteed. It is therefore important to emphasize that the municipality must continue to strive for excellence in coverage, in order to increase access, and at the same time meet the health needs of the user, based on epidemiology, always seeking to balance the supply and demand of its population, guaranteeing continuity of care, and thus achieving Universality with Integrality in oral health.

8 References

AQUILANTE, Aline Guerra; ACIOLE, Geovani Gurgel. Oral health care after the National Oral Health Policy - "Smiling Brazil": a case study. *Ciência & Saùde Coletiva*, v. 20, n. 1, Rio de Janeiro. Jan. 2015, p. 239-48.

BARBOSA, Adrielly Oliveira; GALVÂO, Angélica Haissa; MARTELLI, Petrônio José de Lima. *Oral health in the Family Health Strategy*, 2010.

BARDIN, L. Anàlise de conteùdo Trad. de L.A. Rego e A. Pinheiro. Lisbon: Ediçoes 70, 2006.

BAUER, M.; GASKELL, G. (Orgs.). *Qualitative researching with text, image and sound*. London: Sage, 2008.

BORGHI, Gabriela N. *et al*. Evaluation of the referral and counter-referral system in secondary care in Dentistry. *RFO*, Passo Fundo/RS, v. 18, n. 2, p. 154-59, May/Aug, 2013.

BOTAZZO, C. *Unidade Bàsica de Saùde*: a door to the system revisited. Bauru: EDUSC, 1999.

BRAZIL. *1988 Constitution*. Constitution of the Federative Republic of Brazil. Brasilia/DF: Senado, 1988.

. Ministry of Health. Secretariat of Health Care, Department of Primary Health Care, National Coordination of Oral Health. *Guidelines for the National Oral Health Policy*. Brasilia/DF: Ministry of Health, 2004.

. Ministry of Health. Office of the Minister. *Ordinance No. 1.570, of July 29, 2004*: establishes criteria, norms and requirements for the implantation and qualification of Dental Specialty Centers and Regional Dental Prosthesis Laboratories. Brasilia/DF: Ministry of Health , 2004b. Available Available at: <http://bvsms.saude.gov.br/bvs/saudelegis/gm/2004/prt1570_29_07_2004.html>. Accessed on: 06 Nov. 2015.

. Ministry of Health. Oral Health. *Cadernos de Atençào Bàsica*, n. 17. Brasilia/DF, 2006.

. Ministry of Health. Secretariat of Health Care, Department of Systems Regulation, Evaluation and Control. *Guidelines for the implementation of Regulatory Complexes*. Brasilia/DF: Ministry of Health, 2006a.

. Ministry of Health. Ordinance No. 648. Approves the National Primary Care Policy, establishing revised guidelines and norms for the organization of Primary Care for the Family Health Program (PSF) and the Community Health Agents Program (Pacs). Diàrio Oficial da Uniao, 28 mar. 2006b.

. *Decree No. 7.508 of June 28, 2011.* Regulates Law No. 8.080, of September 19, 1990, to provide for the organization of the Unified Health System - SUS, health planning, health care and inter-federative coordination, and makes other provisions. June 29, 2011. Brasilia/DF: Official Journal of the Union, 2011.

. Ministry of Health. Health Care Secretariat. Health Surveillance Secretariat. *National Oral Health Survey*: main results - SB Brasil 2010. Brasilia/DF, 2012a. Available at: <http://dab.saude.gov.br/portaldab/pnsb.php>. Accessed on: 06 Nov. 2015.

. Ministry of Health. *National Primary Care Policy.* Brasilia: Ministry of Health, 2012b.

BULGARELI, Jaqueline Vilela *et al.* Information from secondary care in Dentistry for evaluating health care models, v. 42, n. 4. *Revista de Odontologia.* UNESP: 2013, p. 229-36.

CAMPOS, G.W.S. *et al.* Reflections on Primary Care and the Family Health Strategy. In: CAMPOS, G.W.S.; GUERREIRO, A.V.P. (Orgs.). *Manual de Pràticas de Atençâo Bàsica.* Sao Paulo: Hucitec, 2010.

CAMPOS, Claudinei José Gomes. Content Analysis: a tool for analyzing qualitative data in the field of health. *Rev Bras Enferm.*, v. 57, n. 5, Sep/Oct 2004, 611-14. Brasilia (DF).

CARVALHO, G. F. P; SPYRIDES, K. S. Prevalence of tooth loss in patients over 50 years of age at the Gama Filho University dental clinic. *Faculdade de Odontologia de Lins/Unimep*, 23(2) 9-16, Jul-Dec, 2013.

CECCIM, Ricardo Burg; FERLA, Alcindo Antônio. Permanent education in health. *Dictionary of permanent health education.* FIOCRUZ, 2009. Available at: <http://www.sites.epsjv.fiocruz.br/dicionario/verbetes/edupersau.html>. Accessed on: July 15, 2016.

CHAVES, Sônia Cristina Lima *et al.* National Oral Health Policy: factors associated with comprehensive care. *Revista Saùde Pùblica*, Salvador/BA, 2010.

CHIZZOTTI, A. *Pesquisa em ciências humanas e sociais.* 8 ed. Sao Paulo: Cortez, 2006.

COSTA, Flâvio Martins da. *Age XEmployability.* Published on 17/09/2007. Available at: <http://www.rh.com.br/Portal/Carreira/Artigo/4848/idade-x-empregabilidade.html>. Accessed on: July 15, 2016.

COSTA, M. A.; COSTA, M. F. B. *Projeto de pesquisa*: entenda e faz. 3 ed. Petrópolis/RJ: Vozes, 2012.

CMS NECKER PINTO. Otics Rio Network. *Internal Regulations.* Available at: <smsdc-cms-

neckerpinto.blogspot.com.br>. Accessed on: 11 Jan. 2016.

CRUZ, M. M. Evaluation of health policies and programs: contributions to the debate. In: MATTOS, R. A.; BAPTISTA, T. W. F. *Caminhospara análise daspoliticas de saù,* 2011, p. 181-99. Available at:<http://www.ims.uerj.br/ccaps/wp-content/uploads/2011/10/Capitulo-7.pdf>. Accessed on: 16 Mar. 2016.

DENZIN, Norman. K.; LINCOLN, Yonna S. *Handbook of qualitative research,* 2nd ed. Thousand Oaks, California: Sage Publications. 2000.

DIAS, A.A. Collective health and legislation in the light of the family health program. IN: DIAS, A. A. *et al. Saùde bucal coletiva*: metodologia de trabalho e pràticas. Sao Paulo: Ed. Santos, 2006, p. 1-20.

ELY, H.C *et al.* Preliminary text, for internal circulation, written to subsidize the preparation of the Cadernos de Atença Bàsica of the Department of Basic Care of the Ministry of Health, volume no. 17, BUCAL HEALTH. Mimeo. Brasilia/Porto Alegre: April 2006. Updated in 2009.

FLEURY, S.; OUVERNEY A.M. *Gestão de redes* : a estratégia de regionalizaçao da política de saù. Rio de Janeiro: FGV, 2007.

FLICK, U. *Introduction to qualitative research.* 3 ed. Translated by J. E. Costa. Sao Paulo: Artmed, 2009.

GIOVANELLA, L.; MENDONÇA, M. H. M. Atençao Primària à Saù. In: GIOVANELLA, L. *et al* (Orgs.). *Health Policies and Systems in Brazil.* Rio de Janeiro: Fiocruz, 2008, p. 575-607.

GIOVANELLA, L. *et al.* Family health: limits and possibilities for a comprehensive approach to primary health care in Brazil. *Ciência & Saùde Coletiva,* v. 14, n. 3, Rio de Janeiro, 2009, p. 783-94.

GONÇALVES, Ingrid Melo *et al.* Progress and results of regulating access to health services in the SUS in Minas Gerais. Published on: 17/03/2010. In: *Consad Congress on Public Management,* 3, 2010, Brasilia. Proceedings. Available at: <http://www.repositorio.fjp.mg.gov.br/consad/handle/123456789/140-pt_br>. Accessed on: 11 Jan. 2016.

GRALHA, R. S.; MORAIS, E. P. PSF in Porto Alegre: socio-historical aspects of implementation. In: LOPES, M. J. M.; PAIXÂO, D. X. *Saùde da familia* : histórias, pràticas e caminhos. Porto Alegre: UFRGS, 2007, p. 31-37.

ODONTO JOURNAL. *Profession.* Year X, n. 151, published on 01/03/2010. Available at:

<http://www.odontomagazine.com.br/2012-05-mulheres-conquistam-a-odontologia-11324>. Accessed on: Mar. 16, 2016.

KUSCHNIR, R.; CHORNY, A. H. Health care networks: contextualizing the debate. *Ciência & Saùde Coletiva*, v. 15, n. 5, Rio de Janeiro, 2010, p. 2307-16. Available at: <http://www.scielo.br/scielo.php?script=sci_arttext&pid=S1413-81232010000500006>. Accessed on: 16 Mar. 2016.

MALTA, D. C. *et al.* Presentation of the strategic action plan for tackling chronic non-communicable diseases in Brazil, 2011 to 2022. *Epidemiol. Serv. Saùde,* v.20 n.4 Brasilia dec. 2011.

MELLO, Ana Lùcia Schaefer Ferreira de. *et al.* Oral health in the care network and the regionalization process. *Ciência & Saùde Coletiva*, v.19, n.1, Rio de Janeiro, 2014, p. 205-14.

MENDES, E.V. *Os grandes dilemas do SUS*. Volume II. Salvador: Casa da Qualidade, 2001.

. Bibliographic review on health care networks. *Minas Gerais State Health Department*. May/2007.

. Health care networks. *Ciência & Saùde Coletiva*, v.15, n.5, 2010, p. 2297-305. Available at: <http://www.scielo.br/pdf/csc/v15n5/v15n5a05>. Accessed on: Mar. 16, 2016.

MINAYO, M.C.S. (Org.). *Pesquisa social*: teoria, método e criatividade. 18 ed. Petrópolis/RJ: Vozes, 2001.

MOYSÉS, Jorge Samuel *et al. Public health*: policies, oral health epidemiology and dental care networks. Sao Paulo: Artes Médicas, 2013. Essential Dentistry Series: interdisciplinary themes.

NARVAI, Paulo Capel. Collective oral health: paths from health dentistry to oral health. *Rev. Saùde Pùblica*, v. 40, n. Especial, 2006, p. 141-47.

NARVAI, Paulo Capel; FRAZÂO, Paulo. *Oral health in Brazil*: far beyond the roof of the mouth. Rio de Janeiro: Fiocruz, 2008 (Coleçao Temas em Saùde).

NAVARRO, Vanessa. Women conquer dentistry. *Odonto*. Published on February 23, 2012. Available at: <http://www.odontomagazine.com.br/2012-05-mulheres- conquistam-a-odontologia-11324>. Accessed on: July 15, 2016.

OLIVEIRA, Maria Amélia de Campos; PEREIRA, Iara Cristina. Essential attributes of Primary Care and the Family Health Strategy. *Rev. Bras. Enfermagem*, v. 66, n. spe, Brasilia, Sep. 2013.

OTICS RIO. *Observatory of information and communication technologies in health systems and services in the city of Rio de Janeiro*. Available at: <www.otics.org>. Accessed on: Jan. 11, 2016.

PIMENTEL, Fernando Castimet *al.* Analysis of oral health care in the Family Health Strategy of

Health District VI, Recife (PE). *Ciência & Saùde Coletiva*, v.15, n.4, Rio de Janeiro, Jul. 2010.

PUGIN, Simone Rossi; NASCIMENTO, Vania Barbosa. *Main milestones of institutional changes in the health sector (1974-1996)*. Didàtica Series, n. 1, Dec. 1996. Available at: <www.cedoc.org.br>. Accessed on: April 17, 2016.

RIO DE JANEIRO. Municipal Health and Civil Defense Secretariat. Primary Care Superintendence. Quick Reference Guide. *Services Portfolio*: list of services provided in Primary Health Care. Municipal Health and Civil Defense Department. Primary Care Superintendence. Rio de Janeiro: SMSDC, 2011. Available at: <http://www.rio.rj.gov.br/dlstatic/10112/137240/DLFE-228987.pdf/1.0>. Accessed on: 06 Nov. 2015.

. *Cadernos de Estatisticas e Mapas da Atençào Primària em Saù do municipio do Rio de Janeiro - CEMAPS RJ*. Jul/2013. Available at:

<http://www.redeoticsrio.org/cmapsrio2013/AP52.html>. Accessed on: 06 Nov. 2015.

. Municipal Health Department. Undersecretariat for Health Promotion, Primary Care and Surveillance, General Health Coordination, Program Area 3.1. *CMS Madre Teresa de Calcutà Internal Regulations*. Published on: 21/08/2015a. Available at: <http://cap31.blogspot.com.br/>. Accessed on: 06 Nov. 2015.

. Municipal Health Secretariat. Undersecretariat for Health Promotion, Primary Care and Surveillance, General Health Coordination, Program Area 3.1 *CMS Parque Royal Internal Regulations.* 2015b. Available at: <http://smsdc-cms-parqueroyal.blogspot.com.br/2015/01/regimento-interno-parque-royal.html>. Accessed on: 06 Nov. 2015.

. Municipal Health and Civil Defense Secretariat. Undersecretariat for Health Promotion, Primary Care and Surveillance - Subpav.; Superintendence for the Integration of Planning Areas - Siape; General Health Coordination for Program Area 3.1 - CGS AP 3.1.*Internal Regulations CF Maria Sebastiana de Oliveira.* 2015c. Available at: <http://smsdc-csf-mariasebastianadeoliveira.blogspot.com.br/>. Accessed on: 06 Nov. 2015.

RODRIGUES, Paulo H.A.; SANTOS, Isabela S. *Saùde e cidadania*: uma visão histórica *e* comparada do SUS. Rio de Janeiro: Atheneu, 2011.

RODRIGUES, Paulo H.A. Desafios politicos para a consolidaçao do Sistema Ùnico de Saùde: uma abordagem histórica. *Hist. Cienc. Saùde-Manguinhos*, v. 21, n. 1, Rio de Janeiro, Jan./Mar. 2014.

SANTOS, A.M.; ASSIS, M.M.A. Da fragmentaçao à integralidade: construindo e (des)construindo a prática de saù oral no Programa de Saù da Familia (PSF) de Alagoinhas, BA. *Ciência & Saùde*

Coletiva, v. 11, n. 1, Rio de Janeiro, 2006, p. 53-61.

SERRA, Carlos Gonçalves. *Guaranteed access to primary care and continuity of care as strategies for consolidating integrality in the SUS*: an analysis of the processes of implementing the PSF, building referral systems and regionalization of care in the state of Rio de Janeiro. 2003. Thesis (Doctorate) - Postgraduate course in Collective Health in Health Policy, Planning and Administration, Institute of Social Medicine, Rio de Janeiro State University (UERJ), Rio de Janeiro, 2003.

SERRA, C.G.; RODRIGUES, P.H.A. Avaliação da referência e contrarreferência no Programa Saùde da Familia na Regiao Metropolitana do Rio de Janeiro (RJ, Brazil). *Ciência & Saùde Coletiva*, v. 15, n. 3, Rio de Janeiro, Nov. 2010.

SILVA, Carlos Letacio Silveira Lessa da. *From the Family Health Program to "Smiling Brazil"*: the road to comprehensiveness in oral health. 2009. Dissertation (Master's Degree) - Faculty of Medicine, Estàcio de Sà University, Rio de Janeiro, 2009.

SILVA, Rodrigo Zouainda. The constitutional right to public health and the integrality of assistance: collision-weighting between the principle of the prohibition of social retrogression and the principle of the reserve of the possible. *Àmbito Juridico*, Rio Grande, v. XIV, n. 95, dec. 2011.

STARFIELD, Barbara. *Primary care*: balancing health needs, services and technology. Brasilia: UNESCO, 2002.

TRIVINOS, A. *Introduction to research in the social sciences*: qualitative research in education. Sao Paulo: Atlas, 1987.

UNICAMP. Department of Oral Diagnosis. Oral Pathology Area. Available at: <w2.fop.unicamp.br/ddo/patologia/downloads/db301>. Accessed on: July 15, 2016.

VERGARA, S.C.. *Research methods in administration*. Sao Paulo: Atlas, 2005.

VILELA, S.M.P. *Relato de experiência*: o problema da fila numa unidade de saù - Recife/PE. 2010. Monograph (Specialization) - Specialization in Management of Health Systems and Services, Ageu Magalhaes Research Center, Osvaldo Cruz Foundation, Recife, 2010.

VILARINHO, S.M.M.; MENDES, R.F.; PRADO JÙNIOR, R.R. Perfil dos cirurgio- dentistas integrantes do Programa Saùde da Familia em Teresina (PI). *Revista Odonto Ciência*, v. 22, n. 55, p. 48-54, 2007.

Appendices

APPENDIX A

UAB INTERVIEW script

Estâcio de Sà University

Masters in Family Health

Research: Challenges for the integration of Oral Health actions between primary and secondary care

in the neighborhood of Ilha do Governador, in the municipality of Rio de Janeiro

BASIC CARE UNIT PROFESSIONALS

Interviewer: ____

Date of interview: _______ / _______ / _______

Block 1 - Professional Profile

Name of interviewee: ____

Unit:

Gender:Male ( ) Female ( )

Age: years

Professional relationship: Permanent ( ) Contracted ( )

If hired, how was it hired?

Workload at this institution:hours

Time since graduation: _______ years

Block 2 - Professional activity

Time working in AB:years

Time working for SUS:years

Have you received training to carry out your work in primary care? ( ) Yes ( ) No.

What do you think about training for dentists in primary care?

Block 3 - Organization and Regulation of Reference and Counter-reference (RCR)

How do you see the ESF in the context of the SUS?

What do you understand by Health Care Networks (HCN)?

In your opinion, how important is the integration of PHC with HCN?

What do you know about comprehensiveness and continuity of care? Are these rights guaranteed by primary care and the CEO? How are they guaranteed?

What dental services does AB provide?

What specialized consultations and exams are offered to primary care patients? Identify the number of professionals provided by the unit for each specialty.

Radiology ( ) ________

Periodontics ( ) ______

Minor oral surgery ( ) _________

Endodontics ( ) ______

Patients with special needs ( ) _______________

Stomatology ( ) ________

Other: ____

Which dental specialties would you include in addition to those provided?

Are you aware of the existence of a clinical protocol for primary care?

( ) Yes ( ) No.

Is it used in your Unit? ( ) Yes ( ) No.

Have you had any training in using the protocol? ( ) Yes ( ) No.

Do you think that referrals to the DSC are made after all the clinical resources in primary care have been exhausted? ( ) Yes ( ) No.

How is access to patients referred from primary care to the CEO regulated?

Point out the three main problems that make it difficult to regulate access to specialties.

1 -

2 -

3 -

How are patients referred from primary care to the CEO monitored?

Do you use any forms to refer patients from the PHC to the CEO?

( ) Yes ( ) No.

Has there been any training for staff in this area? ( ) Yes ( ) No.

Tell the team about the need or importance of this training.

How do you fill in this form (e.g. by hand, scanned)?

Do you think that if filling out the form were digitized, it would bring benefits? Which benefits?

Do you consider the reference form used to be ideal and comprehensive enough? ( ) Yes ( ) No.

What information should be added if it is to be redesigned?

What do you think of the Oral Health RCR System?

Do you work with electronic medical records? ( ) Yes ( ) No. Talk about its importance for the coordination of primary care and the CEO.

What are the specialties with the highest number of referrals? (List three). Identify the average waiting time for each case.

1 - ____

2 - ____

3 - ____

Do you think that the guarantee of access to the secondary level for continuity of care (integrality) is being covered by primary care?

Identify the strengths and weaknesses of access to dental specialties (CEO):

Do the professionals responsible for specialized consultations make counter-referrals? ( ) Yes ( ) No.

Is there a counter-referral form? ( ) Yes ( ) No.

Do you think that the professionals at the CEO fill out this form properly? ( ) Yes ( ) No.

How do you fill in this form (e.g. by hand, scanned)?

Do you think it would be beneficial if the form were digitalized? ( ) Yes ( ) No. Which benefits?

Do you consider the counter-referral form used to be ideal or to contain the necessary information? ( ) Yes ( ) No.

What information should be added if it is to be redesigned?

What is the average turnaround time for patients referred to the CEO for primary care?

Which specialty requires the longest waiting time? How long (on average)?

How does the PC unit behave after the return of the counter-referred patient? Is he scheduled immediately?

Is there a permanent education program for primary care? ( ) Yes ( ) No. Do you think this is important? ( ) Yes ( ) No. Tell us about it.

Is there communication between professionals at the different levels of care? ( ) Yes ( ) No. Is there discussion of the clinical case management of referred patients? ( ) Yes ( ) No. Talk about the importance of this interaction between professionals at the different levels of care.

Is there a plan drawn up by the UABs for referring the most urgent cases? ( ) Yes ( ) No.

What is your opinion on the link between the AB and the CEO?

Is there a regular meeting between the PHC team and the DSC professionals to discuss problems, difficulties and reformulate actions? ( ) Yes ( ) No. If so, how often do these meetings take place? How do you rate this activity?

Is the equipment in the AB unit constantly maintained? ( ) Yes ( ) No. How often?

Is there a lack of supplies to carry out your activities? ( ) Yes ( ) No. What are they?

What is the average waiting time for the necessary materials?

BLOCK 4 - RECOMMENDATIONS

What recommendations do you suggest for improving the network, improving the articulation between primary and secondary care, especially with regard to guaranteeing continuity of care for the user?

END THE INTERVIEW

APPENDIX B

INTERVIEW script - SISREG

Estàcio de Sà University

Family Health Master's Degree

Research: Challenges for the integration of oral health actions between primary and secondary care

in the neighborhood of Ilha do Governador, municipality of Rio de Janeiro

PROFESSIONAL WHO OPERATES SISREG

Interviewer:

Date of interview: _______ / _________ / _________

Block 1 - Professional Profile

Name: ____

Unit:

Gender: Male ( ) Female ( )

Age: years

Employment relationship: Permanent ( ) Contract ( )

If hired, how will you be hired?

Workload at this institution:hours

Training:____

Time since graduation: ________ years

Have you taken any training courses to develop this activity? ( ) Yes ( ) No. Which?

Block 2 - Professional Activity

Function: ____

Time in office: ____________ years

Time working for SUS: ____________years

Have you received specific training for the job? ( ) Yes ( ) No.

Was this training enough for you? ( ) Yes ( ) No. Why not?

Do you think it is important to prepare these professionals for their work? ( ) Yes ( ) No. Why not?

Block 3 - Organization and Regulation of Reference and Counter-reference (RCR)

What do you mean by RAS?

In your opinion, how important is the participation of primary care in the SUS health care network?

How do you see the implementation of CEOS in the process of comprehensive patient care?

Do you think that the oral health clinical protocol is important for referring patients from primary care to the CEO? ( ) Yes ( ) No. Why not?

How do you analyze the offer of specialized consultations and exams for PHC patients in Oral Health?

Are there waiting lists for dental specialties? ( ) Yes ( ) No. If so, how is this monitored?

What specialized consultations and exams are offered to primary care patients? Identify the number of professionals provided by the unit for each specialty.

Radiology ( ) ___________

Periodontics ( ) _________

Minor oral surgery ( ) ___________

Endodontics ( ) _________

Patients with special needs ( ) _________________

Stomatology ( ) ___________

Other: ____

Could you describe the process of regulating vacancies for specialized consultations in BS?

How often does the CEO make vacancies available for specialized services?

Point out the three main problems that make it difficult to regulate access to specialties:

1 -

2 -

3 -

How are patients who have been referred to the CEO from primary care monitored?

What are the criteria used to offer specialized consultations to patients referred by the PC to the CEO?

Is there prioritization between different cases? ( ) Yes ( ) No. What are these priorities?

Which specialties have the highest number of referrals? (List three) Identify the average waiting time for each case.

1 -

2 -

3 -

Do you think that the guarantee of access to the secondary level for continuity of care (integrality) is being covered by primary care when the patient is referred to the CEO? ( ) Yes ( ) No. How?

Identify the strengths and weaknesses of access to dental specialties (CEO):

Do you think that access to specialties is meeting the demands of primary care?

Are referrals made using specific forms? ( ) Yes ( ) No.

Are these forms always filled in properly? ( ) Yes ( ) No.

Are there any specific criteria for filling specialized vacancies? ( ) Yes ( ) No.

Is there any training for the team in this area? ( ) Yes ( ) No. Tell us about the need or importance of this training for the team.

How do I fill in this form (e.g. by hand, digitally)?

Do you think it would be beneficial if the form were digitalized? ( ) Yes ( ) No. Which benefits?

Have you ever discussed introducing electronic medical records for this purpose? ( ) Yes ( ) No.

Do you consider the reference form used to be ideal and provide the necessary information? ( ) Yes ( ) No.

What information should always be included in the form? From your experience, do you suggest anything that could be added?

Block 4 - Communication and information resources

Is there communication between the professionals at the PC unit and the regulatory system (SISREG)?

( ) Yes ( ) No.

What communication resources are available in the units? AB, SISREG and CEO.

( ) Computer connected to a network;

( ) Computer not connected to the network;

( ) Telephone;

( ) Radio (or Nextel type).

Do all units have these resources available? ( ) Yes ( ) No.

Does the vacancy regulation system respond to the demands of primary care DCs? ( ) Yes ( ) No.

Does this fall within the regulatory remit? ( ) Yes ( ) No.

How do you see this communication?

What are the means used for referrals and counter-referrals in the Basic Units?

AB and CEO.

( ) Paper guide;

( ) Telephone/radio;

( ) Computer network guidance.

How are the RCR forms filled in (e.g. by hand, scanned)?

Would it benefit you to digitize the form? ( ) Yes ( ) No. Which benefits?

BLOCK 5 - RECOMMENDATIONS

What recommendations do you have for improving or speeding up the regulation of vacancies for the secondary level in Oral Health?

END THE INTERVIEW

APPENDIX C

INTERVIEW script - CEO

Estâcio de Sà University
Family Health Master's Degree
Research: Challenges for the integration of Oral Health actions between primary and secondary care
and secondary care in the neighborhood of Ilha do Governador, in the municipality of Rio de Janeiro

<u>**CEO PROFESSIONALS**</u>

Interviewer: ____

Date of interview: _______ / _________ / _________

Block 1 - Professional profile

Name: ____

Unit:

Gender: Male ( ) Female ( )

Age: years

Professional relationship: Permanent ( ) Contracted ( )

If hired, how will you be hired?

Workload at this institution:hours

Time since graduation: _________ years

What is the CEO's specialty? _______________________________________

Do you have a specialization course in the dental specialty in which you work at the CEO? ( ) Yes (

) No.

Can you develop all your professional skills at CEO?

( ) Yes ( ) No. What do you think is missing?

Block 2 - Professional activity

Time at CEO: _____________________ years

Time working in the specialty: _______________ years

Time working for SUS: _____________ years

Have you received training to perform your duties at the CEO? ( ) Yes ( ) No.

Do you think training is important? ( ) Yes ( ) No. Why not?

Block 3 - Organization and Regulation of Reference and Counter-reference (RCR)

How do you see the ESF in the context of the SUS?

What do you understand by Health Care Networks (HCN)?

How do you understand the HCN based on primary care?

In your opinion, how important is the CEO in the SAN?

How do you understand the principle of integrality (in the sense of continuity of care)? Are these rights guaranteed by the CEO? ( ) Yes ( ) No. How?

How do you schedule patients at your health unit? What are the main difficulties you perceive in scheduling patients?

Are specialized consultations and exams available to meet the needs of patients at the Primary Care Unit? ( ) Yes ( ) No.

How do you offer appointments for specialties at the CEO?

Do you have any criteria for organizing your vacancies? ( ) Yes ( ) No. Which criteria?

What specialized consultations and exams are offered to primary care patients? Identify the number of professionals provided by the unit for each specialty.

Radiology ( ) ________

Periodontics ( ) ______

Minor oral surgery ( ) _________

Endodontics ( ) ______

Patients with special needs ( ) _______________

Stomatology ( ) ________

Other: ____

What criteria are used to offer specialized consultations to patients referred by the PC to the CEO?

Is there prioritization between different cases? ( ) Yes ( ) No.

Do you think this number of professionals is sufficient? ( ) Yes ( ) No.

Why?

How is access to patients referred from the PA to the CEO regulated?

Do CEO professionals receive institutional support to clarify doubts?

( ) Yes ( ) No.

What criteria are used to offer appointments to Network patients?

Do patients referred to the DSC by the PC arrive with the referral forms filled in properly? ( ) Yes ( ) No. What are the most common errors?

Name the three main problems that make it difficult to regulate referrals for consultations and exams:

1 -

2 -

3 -

Do you keep a statistical record of the demand for your specialty?

Do you have a communication channel with the AB CDs?

What are the most popular specialties? (List three).

Identify the average waiting time in each case.

1 -

2 -

3 -

What criteria are used to offer specialized consultations to patients referred by the PC to the CEO?
Are there any priority criteria for specialized care? ( ) Yes ( ) No. Which criteria?

Do you think that guaranteeing access to the secondary level for continuity of care (integrality) is meeting the demands of primary care? ( ) Yes ( ) No. How?

Identify the strengths and weaknesses of access to dental specialties (CEO):

How are counter-referrals handled? Is there a protocol/form to be used?

Are the forms always filled in? ( ) Yes ( ) No.

Did you notice any difficulties in filling it in? ( ) Yes ( ) No. Which ones?

What recommendations are given to patients who are counter-referred to PHC? Are there any special recommendations? ( ) Yes ( ) No. In what situations?

Is there any training in this area? ( ) Yes ( ) No. Tell us about the need or importance of this training for the team.

How do you fill in this form (e.g. by hand, scanned)?

Do you think it would be beneficial if the form were digitalized? ( ) Yes ( ) No.

Which ones? ____

Do you think the counter-referral form used is ideal and contains the necessary information? What information could be added?

How do you understand the role of CEO professionals in comprehensive oral health care?

Do you work with electronic medical records? ( ) Yes ( ) No. Please comment on their importance for the coordination of primary care and the CEO.

Is there a continuing education program for the CEO? ( ) Yes ( ) No. Do you think this is important? ( ) Yes ( ) No. Tell us about it.

Is there communication between professionals at the different levels of care? ( ) Yes ( ) No. Is there discussion of the clinical case management of referred patients? ( ) Yes ( ) No. Talk about the importance of this interaction between professionals at the different levels of care.

How do you assess the link between the PC and the CEO?

Is there a regular meeting between the PA team and the CEO professionals to discuss problems, difficulties and reformulate actions? ( ) Yes ( ) No. If so, how often do these meetings take place? How do you analyze this activity?

Is the CEO's equipment constantly maintained? ( ) Yes ( ) No.

Is there a lack of supplies for specialized activities? ( ) Yes ( ) No. What are they?

What is the average waiting time for the necessary materials?

BLOCK 4 - RECOMMENDATIONS

What recommendations do you have for improving the interaction between BAs and CEOs?

END THE INTERVIEW

APPENDIX D

INTERVIEW script - ORAL HEALTH COORDINATOR

Estàcio de Sà University

Family Health Master's Degree

Research: Challenges for the integration of Oral Health actions between primary and secondary care

and secondary care in the neighborhood of Ilha do Governador, in the municipality of Rio de Janeiro

<u>**ORAL HEALTH COORDINATOR/COORDINATION**</u>

Interviewer:

Date of interview: _______ / _______ / _________

Block 1 - Professional Profile

Name of interviewee: ____

Unit:

Gender: Male ( ) Female ( )

Age: years

Employment relationship: Permanent ( ) Contract ( )

If hired, how will you be hired?

Workload at this institution:hours

Time since graduation: _______ years

Block 2 - Professional Activity

Position: ____

Time in office: _________ years

Time working for SUS:years

Have you received training to perform your job? ( ) Yes ( ) No.

Was this training enough for you? ( ) Yes ( ) No. Why not?

Do you consider these trainings important? ( ) Yes ( ) No. Which ones would you like to have?

Block 3 - Organization and Regulation of Reference and Counter-reference (RCR)

How is the supply of specialized consultations and exams planned to guarantee the demand of UAB patients?

How is the supply of specialized consultations and exams sized (programmed)?

Have referrals been made based on protocols? ( ) Yes ( ) No. Which protocols are in use?

Are PHC and DSC professionals aware of the protocol/form established for patients' RCR? ( ) Yes ( ) No.

Are these professionals trained in the use of protocols/forms?

( ) Yes ( ) No.

How often does this training take place? _______________________________

Is there an evaluation of the use of the protocols? ( ) Yes ( ) No.

Are PHC and DSC professionals supported in relation to doubts or difficulties in CRR? ( ) Yes ( ) No. How is this support provided?

How is oral health regulated?

Name the three main problems that make it difficult to regulate referrals for consultations and exams:

1 -

2 -

3 -

Are there any initiatives to improve/make more agile the regulation of vacancies in SB?

Are queues monitored? ( ) Yes ( ) No. How is this problem dealt with?

What are the specialties with the highest number of referrals? (List three). Identify the average waiting time for each case.

1 -

2 -

3 -

Do you think the number of professionals at the CEO is sufficient?

( ) Yes ( ) No. Justify and give examples. How do you intend to solve the question?

Do you think that the current state of regulation is guaranteeing continuity of care (integrality)? ( ) Yes ( ) No. Why not?

What is the turnaround time for patients referred to the CEO? Is there any initiative to speed up counter-referral? ( ) Yes ( ) No.

Are there any rules in place to ensure that the counter-referred patient is quickly scheduled for further care? ( ) Yes ( ) No. What is it?

Are there any rules governing communication between professionals at different levels of care? ( ) Yes ( ) No.

Do you think there is a link between primary care and the CEO? ( ) Yes ( ) No.

What do you think of the importance of this articulation?

Block 4 - Communication and Information Resources

Do the units work with electronic patient records? ( ) Yes ( ) No. How important is it? Are there any plans for its implementation?

Is there a means of communication between the professionals at the primary care unit and the CEO? ( ) Yes ( ) No. What means do you use or what are they?

What communication resources are available in the units?

( ) Computer connected to a network;

( ) Computer not connected to the network;

( ) Telephone;

( ) Radio (or Nextel type).

Do all units have these resources available? ( ) Yes ( ) No. What means are used for referrals and counter-referrals?

( ) Paper guide;

( ) Telephone/radio;

( ) Computer network guidance.

How are the RCR forms filled in (e.g. by hand, scanned)?

Would it benefit you to digitize the form?( ) Yes ( ) No. Which benefits?

Block 5 - Logistics

Is there planning for the supply of medicines, supplies and materials used in consultations or specialized SB exams? ( ) Yes ( ) No.

Is there stock control? ( ) Yes ( ) No.

Have there been any shortages of medication, supplies, instruments or equipment?

( ) Yes ( ) No. If so, what are the main items that have been missing?

Is the equipment used regularly maintained and calibrated? ( ) Yes ( ) No. What is the average waiting time for the necessary materials?

Block 6 - Recommendations

What are the recommendations/initiatives for improving the link between primary and secondary oral health care?

END THE INTERVIEW

APPENDIX E

INFORMED CONSENT FORM (TCLE - UNESA)

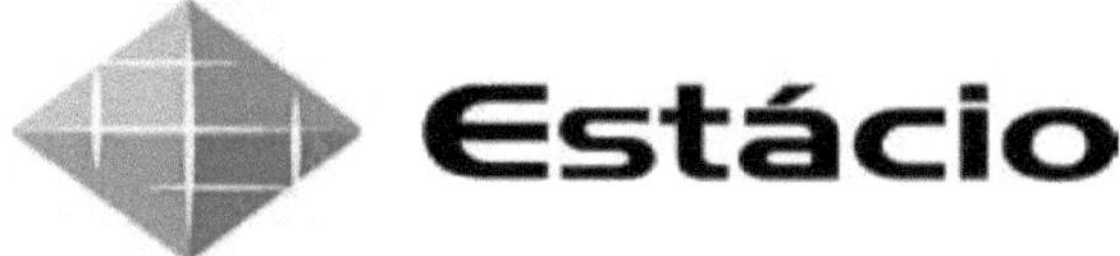

MANDATORY INFORMED CONSENT FORM

FOR SCIENTIFIC RESEARCH ON HUMAN BEINGS

<u>**Identification data of the research participant**</u>:

Name: ____

Gender: Male ( ) Female ( ) Date of Birth: _________________ / _____ / _________

Address: ____

Neighborhood: _________________________________ City: ________________________

Phone: (_____) ________________________

Email: ____

<u>**Title of Research Protocol**</u>: Challenges for the integration of Oral Health actions between primary and secondary care in the neighborhood of Ilha do Governador, Rio de Janeiro.

Research Sub-Area: Family Health Practices and Technologies

Researcher responsible: Luciana da Silva Oliveira Gomes

Institution: Universidade Estàcio de Sà - UNESA - Campus Arcos da Lapa/RJ

Address: Rua Riachuelo, 27. ZIP CODE: 20230-010

Phone: (21) 99968-5899 / E-mail: rj.lugomes@gmail.com

Advisor: Prof. Dr. Carlos Gonçalves Serra

Tel: (21) 98898-9150 / E-mail: carlosgser@gmail.com

Research Ethics Committee: Tel: (21) 2215-1485

E-mail: cepsms@rio.rj.gov.br / Hours: Tuesday to Friday, 9 a.m. to 4 p.m.

Research risk assessment:

 (X) Minimum Risk ( ) Medium Risk ( ) Low Risk ( ) Higher Risk

Objectives:

General: To analyze how the articulation between primary and secondary care takes place with regard to oral health actions in the district of Ilha do Governador, in the municipality of Rio de Janeiro.

Specifics:

• To describe the offer of oral health services in secondary care used by primary care units in the Zumbi and Bancàrios neighborhoods;

• To analyze the criteria adopted by dental surgeons to refer users registered at the Zumbi and Bancàrios units to the secondary unit;

• Describe how scheduling for specialized oral health appointments works;

• Know the counter-referral flow from the Specialty Center

Dental Center (CEO);

• Identify the strengths and weaknesses of access to dental specialties.

Justification:

The initial motivation for the research was due to the researcher's concern about the constant complaints from patients when they were referred to the Dental Specialties Center (CEO), due to the difficulty in scheduling appointments via the vacancy regulation system. This gave rise to a concern to study how the articulation between the primary and secondary levels of care is taking place in everyday practice. To this end, it is essential to analyze the referral and counter-referral system, which is considered an important tool created and used by the SUS to guarantee continuity of oral health care. It is hoped that the results of this study will provide important elements for improving clinical management and user care in order to take account of their right to health and comprehensiveness, as advocated by the SUS.

Procedures:

Participation consists of answering an interview (or questionnaire) about what you know about the aforementioned project. This instrument will be presented to you if you agree to take part in this research.

Risks and inconveniences:

It is considered a study with minimal risk for the participants, i.e. they can be involved in activities such as talking, walking or reading.

Potential benefits:

It is hoped that the results of this study will provide important elements for reviewing the daily practice of the referral and counter-referral system and contribute to improving clinical management and user care in order to fulfill their right to health and comprehensiveness, as advocated by the SUS.

Additional Information:

If you have any considerations or doubts about the ethics of the research, you can contact the Research Ethics Committee (CEP) of the Estàcio de Sà University, during business hours, by e-mail: cep.unesa@estacio.br or by telephone: (21) 3231-6139.

For this research, there will be no cost to the participant at any stage of the study. Likewise, there will be no financial compensation related to your participation. You will have full and complete freedom to refuse to participate or to withdraw your consent at any stage of the research.

I believe that I have been sufficiently informed about the information that I have read or that has been read to me, describing the study: "Challenges for the integration of Oral Health actions between primary and secondary care in the neighborhood of Ilha do Governador, municipality of Rio de Janeiro". The purpose of this research is clear. Likewise, I am aware of the procedures to be carried out, their discomforts and risks, the guarantees of confidentiality and ongoing clarification. It is also clear that my participation is free of charge. I voluntarily agree to my participation, knowing that I can withdraw my consent at any time, before or during the procedure, without penalty or prejudice. This form will be signed in two copies of equal content, one for the research participant and one for the person responsible for the research.

Rio de Janeiro, ______________/ ________________ / ________ .

Signature of Research Participant: ____

Signature of the person responsible for the research:

Annexes

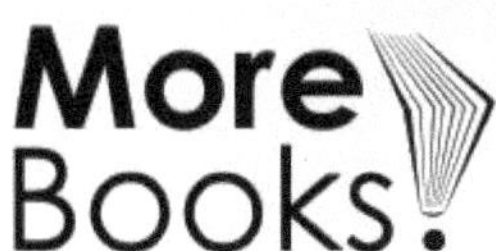

More
Books!

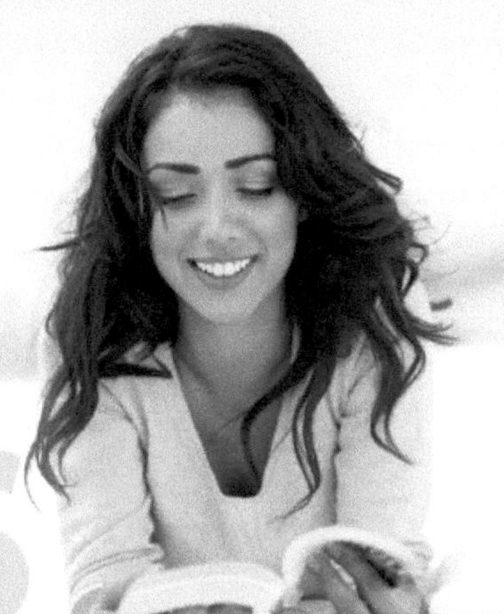

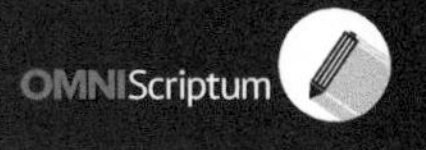

info@omniscriptum.com
www.omniscriptum.com
OMNIScriptum

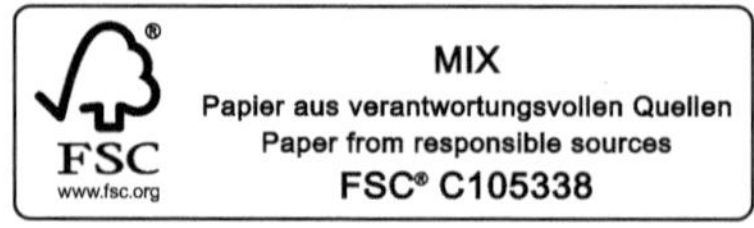

Printed by Books on Demand GmbH, Norderstedt / Germany